PARTIAL SOLUTIONS MANUAL

to accompany

INTERMEDIATE ALGEBRA
For College Students,
Third Edition

Jerome E. Kaufmann

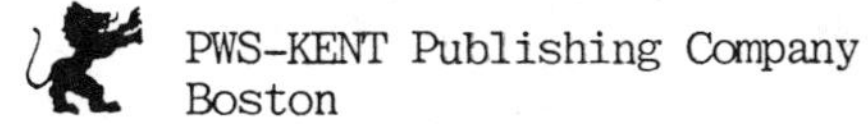

PWS–KENT Publishing Company
Boston

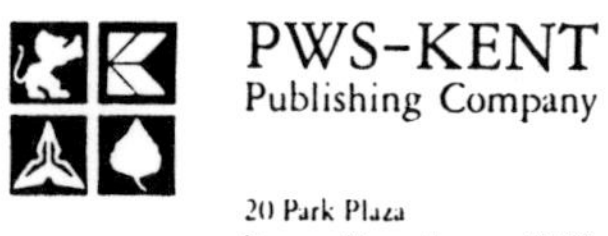

PWS-KENT
Publishing Company

20 Park Plaza
Boston, Massachusetts 02116

Printed in the United States of America.

91 92 93 - 10 9 8 7 6 5 4

ISBN 0-534-91623-6

PREFACE

This student supplement has been prepared to accompany the <u>Third Edition</u> <u>of</u> <u>Intermediate</u> <u>Algebra</u> <u>for</u> <u>College</u> <u>Students</u>. Detailed solutions for approximately one-fourth of the exercises are included. In general, we have included the solutions for problems numbered 1, 5, 9, 13, and so on. If such problems are short-answer problems with no work to be shown, however, they have occasionally not been included since the answers are in the back of the text.

Certainly many of the exercises can be solved in different ways. In order to keep this supplement a reasonable size, we have usually shown only one approach to a problem. Therefore, you may use an approach which is different and perhaps simpler than the way shown. However, if you cannot solve a problem, then referring to our suggestions should be of some help. It is to your advantage to use this supplement only after you have made a sincere effort to solve the problem by yourself.

Good luck in your study of intermediate algebra.

J. Kaufmann

CONTENTS

Chapter 1

Problem Set 1.1

1. This is a true statement because the real numbers consist of the rationals and irrationals.

5. This is a true statement because every integer can be expressed as the indicated quotient of two integers. For example, $6 = \frac{6}{1}$.

9. This is a true statement because the set of whole numbers is a subset of the set of integers.

13. The numbers 0, 14, $\frac{2}{3}$, $-\frac{11}{14}$, 2.34, $3.2\overline{1}$, $6\frac{7}{8}$, -19, and -2.6 are all rational numbers.

17. All of the numbers in the list are real numbers.

21. Every integer is a rational number.

25. Every natural number is a whole number.

29. Every odd number is an integer.

33. The set of natural numbers consists of $\{1,2,3,4,\dots\}$; therefore, the set described is $\{1,2\}$.

37. The set of integers is $\{\dots-2,-1,0,1,2,\dots\}$; therefore, the set described is $\{-1,0,1,2\}$.

41. The set of nonnegative integers is $\{0,1,2,3,\dots\}$; therefore, the set described is $\{0,1,2,3,4\}$.

45. Substituting 2 for n, the statement $3n+4 = 7$ becomes $3(2)+4 = 7$. The statement $3(2)+4 = 7$ is false but that is not the issue here.

49. The reflexive property states that $a = a$ for any real number $\underline{a}$. Therefore, the statement $5x = 5x$ can be made.

53. Do the multiplications and divisions in the order that they appear from left to right.
$$9 \div 3 \cdot 4 \div 2 \cdot 14 = 3 \cdot 4 \div 2 \cdot 14 = 12 \div 2 \cdot 14 = 6 \cdot 14 = 84$$

57. Do the multiplications first. Then do the additions and subtractions in the order that they appear from left to right.
$$9 \cdot 7 - 4 \cdot 5 - 3 \cdot 2 + 4 \cdot 7 = 63 - 20 - 6 + 28 = 43 - 6 + 28 = 37 + 28 = 65$$

61. Do the subtractions inside the parentheses first. Then multiply and then add.
$$13 + (7-2)(5-1) = 13 + (5)(4) = 13 + 20 = 33$$

65. Work from the inside out on the parentheses and brackets.
$$7[3(6-2)] - 64 = 7[3(4)] - 64 = 7(12) - 64 = 84 - 64 = 20$$

69. Work inside the parentheses first. Then multiply and then add and subtract.
$$14 + 4\left(\frac{8-2}{12-9}\right) - 2\left(\frac{9-1}{19-15}\right) = 14 + 4\left(\frac{6}{3}\right) - 2\left(\frac{8}{4}\right) = 14 + 4(2) - 2(2) = 14 + 8 - 4 = 18$$

73. Work above and below the horizontal bar first.
$$\frac{3 \cdot 8 - 4 \cdot 3}{5 \cdot 7 - 34} + 19 = \frac{24-12}{35-34} + 19 = \frac{12}{1} + 19 = 12 + 19 = 31$$

<u>Problem Set 1.2</u>

1. $(-6)+(-9) = -(|-6|+|-9|) = -(6+9) = -15$

5. $12+(-3) = |12|-|-3| = 12-3 = 9$

9. $-12-9 = -12+(-9) = -(|-12|+|-9|) = -21$

13. $14-(-10) = 14+10 = 24$

17. $19+(-31) = -(|-31|-|19|) = -(31-19) = -12$

21. $17-36 = 17+(-36) = -(|-36|-|17|) = -(36-17) = -19$

25. $63+(-34) = |63|-|-34| = 63-34 = 29$

29. $-47-(-56) = -47+56 = |56|-|-47| = 56-47 = 9$

33. $|-34|-|-62| = 34-62 = 34+(-62) = -28$

37. $|6+(-10)| = |-4| = 4$

41. $9-12-8+5-6 = 9+(-12)+(-8)+5+(-6) = -12$

45. $12+(-14)+16-(-11)+9 = 12+(-14)+16+11+9 = 34$

49. $-6-8-10-16-4 = -6+(-8)+(-10)+(-16)+(-4) = -44$

53. $(6-8)-(7+2) = (-2)-9 = -2+(-9) = -11$

57. $16-18+19-[14-22-(31-41)] = 16-18+19-[14-22-(-10)]$
$$= 16-18+19-[14-22+10] = 16-18+19-[2] = 15$$

<u>Problem Set 1.3</u>

1. $(-8)(-5) = |-8|\cdot|-5| = 8\cdot5 = 40$

5. $(-5)(13) = -(|-5|\cdot|13|) = -(5\cdot13) = -65$

9. $(-81)\div3 = -(81\div3) = -27$ 13. $(-4)(-3)(6) = 12(6) = 72$

17. $(9)(-3)(2) = (-27)(2) = -54$ 21. Division by zero is undefined.

25. $(-16)\div(-2)\div(-4) = 8\div(-4) = -2$ 29. $-(\frac{-12}{4}) = -(-3) = 3$

33. $6-(5)(-3) = 6-(-15) = 6+15 = 21$

37. $5(-6)-(-4)(11) = -30-(-44) = -30+44 = 14$

41. $3(5-9)-(3)(-6) = 3(-4)-(-18) = -12+18 = 6$

45. $-6(-3-9-1) = (-6)(-13) = 78$

49. $-3[5-(-2)]-2(-4-9) = (-3)(7)-2(-13) = -21+26 = 5$

53. $[(-3)(4)-(-2)(1)][(-2)(-7)-(-8)(6)] = [-12+2][14+48] = (-10)(62) = -620$

57. $(-7-5)(6-10)-(2-7)(-3-2)+11 = (-12)(-4)-(-5)(-5)+11 = 48-25+11 = 34$

<u>Problem Set 1.4</u>

17. $[83+(-99)]+18 = -16+18 = 2$ 21. $17(97)+17(3) = 17(97+3)$
$$= 17(100) = 1700$$

25. $(-50)(15)(-2)-(-4)(17)(25) = 100(15)-(-100)(17) = 1500+1700 = 3200$

29. $-5^2-4^2 = -25-16 = -41$

33. $3(-1)^3-4(3)^2 = 3(-1)-4(9) = -3-36 = -39$

37. $-3-(-2)^3+4(-1)^5 = -3(-8)+4(-1) = 24-4 = 20$

41. $2^3+3(-1)^3(-2)^2-5(-1)(2)^2 = 8+3(-1)(4)-5(-1)(4) = 8-12+20 = 16$

45. $[3(-2)^2-2(-3)^2]^3 = [3(4)-2(9)]^3 = [12-18]^3 = (-6)^3 = -216$

49. $2^4-2(2)^3-3(2)^2+7(2)-10 = 16-2(8)-3(4)+14-10 = 16-16-12+14-10 = -8$

<u>Problem Set 1.5</u>

1. $-7x+11x = (-7+11)x = 4x$ 5. $4n-9n-n = (4-9-1)n = -6n$

9. $-3a^2+7b^2+9a^2-2b^2 = (-3+9)a^2+(7-2)b^2 = 6a^2+5b^2$

13. $5a^2b-ab^2-7a^2b = (5-7)a^2b-ab^2 = -2a^2b-ab^2$

17. $-2(a-4)-3(a+2) = -2a+8-3a-6 = -5a+2$

21. $-6(x^2-5)-(x^2-2) = -6x^2+30-x^2+2 = -7x^2+32$

25. $3(2x-5)-4(5x-2) = 6x-15-20x+8 = -14x-7$

29. $3(2x-4y)-2(x+9y) = 6x-12y-2x-18y = 4x-30y$

33. $-(3x-1)-2(5x-1)+4(-2x-3) = -3x+1-10x+2-8x-12 = -21x-9$

37. $4x^2-y^2 = 4(2)^2-(-2)^2 = 4(4)-4 = 16-4 = 12$

41. $2x^2-4xy-3y^2 = 2(1)^2-4(1)(-1)-3(-1)^2 = 2(1)+4-3(1) = 2+4-3 = 3$

45. $7a-2b-9a+3b = -2a+b = -2(4)+(-6) = -8-6 = -14$

49. $-2a-3a+7b-b = -5a+6b = -5(-10)+6(9) = 50+54 = 104$

53. $2(x-1)-(x+2)-3(2x-1) = 2x-2-x-2-6x+3 = -5x-1 = -5(-1)-1 = 5-1 = 4$

57. $5(x-2y)-3(2x+y)-2(x-y) = 5x-10y-6x-3y-2x+2y = -3x-11y = -3(-1)-11(-2)$
$$= 3+22 = 25$$

Chapter 2

<u>Problem Set 2.1</u>

1. $3x+4 = 16$
    $3x = 12$ Add -4 to both sides.
    $x = 4$ Multiply both sides by $\frac{1}{3}$.

The solution set is $\{4\}$.

5. $-x-6 = 8$
    $-x = 14$ Add 6 to both sides.
    $x = -14$ Multiply both sides by -1.

The solution set is $\{-14\}$.

9. $3x-4 = 15$
    $3x = 19$ Add 4 to both sides.
    $x = \frac{19}{3}$ Multiply both sides by $\frac{1}{3}$.

The solution set is $\{\frac{19}{3}\}$.

13. $-6y-4 = 16$
    $-6y = 20$ Add 4 to both sides.
    $y = -\frac{20}{6}$ Multiply both sides by $-\frac{1}{6}$.
    $y = -\frac{10}{3}$ Reduce.

The solution set is $\{-\frac{10}{3}\}$.

17. $5y+2 = 2y-11$
    $3y+2 = -11$ Add -2y to both sides.
    $3y = -13$ Add -2 to both sides.
    $y = -\frac{13}{3}$ Multiply both sides by $\frac{1}{3}$.

The solution set is $\{-\frac{13}{3}\}$.

21. $-7a+6 = -8a+14$
    $a+6 = 14$ Add 8a to both sides.
    $a = 8$ Add -6 to both sides.

The solution set is $\{8\}$.

25. $6y+18+y = 2y+3$
    $7y+18 = 2y+3$ Combine similar terms.
    $5y+18 = 3$ Add -2y to both sides.
    $5y = -15$ Add -18 to both sides.
    $y = -3$ Multiply both sides by $\frac{1}{5}$.

The solution set is $\{-3\}$.

29. $6n-4-3n = 3n+10+4n$

    $3n-4 = 7n+10$ Combine similar terms on both sides.

      $-4 = 4n+10$ Add $-3n$ to both sides.

    $-14 = 4n$ Add -10 to both sides.

    $-\dfrac{14}{4} = n$ Multiply both sides by $\dfrac{1}{4}$.

    $-\dfrac{7}{2} = n$ Reduce.

The solution set is $\{-\dfrac{7}{2}\}$.

33. $-3(x-2) = 11$

    $-3x+6 = 11$ Apply distributive property.

      $-3x = 5$ Add -6 to both sides.

        $x = -\dfrac{5}{3}$ Multiply both sides by $-\dfrac{1}{3}$.

The solution set is $\{-\dfrac{5}{3}\}$.

37. $5x-4(x-6) = -11$

    $5x-4x+24 = -11$ Apply distributive property.

       $x+24 = -11$ Combine similar terms.

           $x = -35$ Add -24 to both sides.

The solution set is $\{-35\}$.

41. $-2(3x+5) = 3(4x+3)$

    $-6x-10 = -12x-9$ Apply distributive property on both sides.

      $6x-10 = -9$ Add $12x$ to both sides.

        $6x = 1$ Add 10 to both sides.

         $x = \dfrac{1}{6}$ Multiply both sides by $\dfrac{1}{6}$.

The solution set is $\{\dfrac{1}{6}\}$.

45. $-2(3n-1)+3(n+5) = -4(n-4)$

    $-6n+2+3n+15 = -4n+16$ Apply distributive property.

        $-3n+17 = -4n+16$ Combine similar terms.

          $n+17 = 16$ Add $4n$ to both sides.

             $n = -1$ Add -17 to both sides.

The solution set is $\{-1\}$.

49. $-2(n-4)-(3n-1) = -2+(2n-1)$

    $-2n+8-3n+1 = -2+2n-1$ Apply distributive property.

        $-5n+9 = 2n-3$ Combine similar terms.

          $9 = 7n-3$ Add $5n$ to both sides.

        $12 = 7n$

       $\dfrac{12}{7} = n$ Multiply both sides by $\dfrac{1}{7}$.

The solution set is $\{\dfrac{12}{7}\}$.

53. Let n represent the smallest integer. Then n+1 and n+2 represent the next
    two consecutive integers.

$$n+(n+1)+(n+2) = 42$$
$$3n+3 = 42$$
$$3n = 39$$
$$n = 13$$

The integers are 13, 14, and 15.

57. Let n represent the smaller number. Then 6n-3 represents the larger
    number. Subtracting the smaller from the larger produces 67.

$$(6n-3)-n = 67$$
$$5n-3 = 67$$
$$5n = 70$$
$$n = 14$$

The numbers are 14 and 6(14)-3 = 81.

61. Let p represent the number of pennies. Then 2p-10 represents the number
    of nickels and 3p-20 represents the number of dimes.

$$p+(2p-10)+(3p-20) = 150$$
$$6p-30 = 150$$
$$6p = 180$$
$$p = 30$$

Maria has 30 pennies, 2(30)-10 = 50 nickels, and 3(30)-20 = 70 dimes.

65. Let x represent the number of three-bedroom apartments. Then 3x+10 and
    6x+20 represent the number of two-bedroom and one-bedroom apartments,
    respectively.

$$x+(3x+10)+(6x+20) = 230$$
$$10x+30 = 230$$
$$10x = 200$$
$$x = 20$$

There are 20, 3(20)+10 = 70, and 6(20)+20 = 140 three-bedroom, two-bedroom,
and one-bedroom apartments, respectively.

Problem Set 2.2

1. $$\frac{3}{4}x = 9$$

$$\frac{4}{3}\left(\frac{3}{4}x\right) = \frac{4}{3}(9) \qquad \text{Multiply both sides by } \frac{4}{3}.$$
$$x = 12$$

The solution set is {12}.

5. $$\frac{n}{2} - \frac{2}{3} = \frac{5}{6}$$

$$6\left(\frac{n}{2} - \frac{2}{3}\right) = 6\left(\frac{5}{6}\right) \qquad \text{Multiply both sides by 6.}$$
$$3n-4 = 5$$
$$3n = 9$$
$$n = 3$$

The solution set is {3}.

9. $$\frac{a}{4} - 1 = \frac{a}{3} + 2$$

$12(\frac{a}{4} - 1) = 12(\frac{a}{3} + 2)$ Multiply both sides by 12.

$$3a - 12 = 4a + 24$$
$$-36 = a$$

The solution set is $\{-36\}$.

13. $$\frac{h}{2} - \frac{h}{3} + \frac{h}{6} = 1$$

$6(\frac{h}{2} - \frac{h}{3} + \frac{h}{6}) = 6(1)$ Multiply both sides by 6.

$$3h - 2h + h = 6$$
$$2h = 6$$
$$h = 3$$

The solution set is $\{3\}$.

17. $$\frac{x+2}{2} - \frac{x-1}{5} = \frac{3}{5}$$

$10(\frac{x+2}{2} - \frac{x-1}{5}) = 10(\frac{3}{5})$ Multiply both sides by 10.

$$5(x+2) - 2(x-1) = 6$$
$$5x + 10 - 2x + 2 = 6$$
$$3x + 12 = 6$$
$$3x = -6$$
$$x = -2$$

The solution set is $\{-2\}$.

21. $$\frac{y}{3} + \frac{y-5}{10} = \frac{4y+3}{5}$$

$$30(\frac{y}{3} + \frac{y-5}{10}) = 30(\frac{4y+3}{5})$$
$$10y + 3(y-5) = 6(4y+3)$$
$$10y + 3y - 15 = 24y + 18$$
$$13y - 15 = 24y + 18$$
$$-33 = 11y$$
$$-3 = y$$

The solution set is $\{-3\}$.

25. $$\frac{2x-1}{8} - 1 = \frac{x+5}{7}$$

$$56(\frac{2x-1}{8} - 1) = 56(\frac{x+5}{7})$$
$$7(2x-1) - 56 = 8(x+5)$$
$$14x - 7 - 56 = 8x + 40$$
$$14x - 63 = 8x + 40$$
$$6x = 103$$
$$x = \frac{103}{6}$$

The solution set is $\{\frac{103}{6}\}$.

29. $$x + \frac{3x-1}{9} - 4 = \frac{3x+1}{3}$$

$$9(x + \frac{3x-1}{9} - 4) = 9(\frac{3x+1}{3})$$
$$9x + 3x - 1 - 36 = 3(3x+1)$$
$$12x - 37 = 9x + 3$$
$$3x = 40$$
$$x = \frac{40}{3}$$

The solution set is $\{\frac{40}{3}\}$.

33. $$n + \frac{2n-3}{9} - 2 = \frac{2n+1}{3}$$

$$9(n + \frac{2n-3}{9} - 2) = 9(\frac{2n+1}{3})$$
$$9n + 2n - 3 - 18 = 3(2n+1)$$
$$11n - 21 = 6n + 3$$
$$5n = 24$$
$$n = \frac{24}{5}$$

The solution set is $\{\frac{24}{5}\}$.

37. $\quad \frac{1}{2}(2x-1) -\frac{1}{3}(5x+2) = 3$

$6[\frac{1}{2}(2x-1) -\frac{1}{3}(5x+2)] = 6(3)$

$3(2x-1)-2(5x+2) = 18$

$6x-3-10x-4 = 18$

$-4x-7 = 18$

$-4x = 25$

$x = -\frac{25}{4}$

The solution set is $\{-\frac{25}{4}\}$.

41. Let n represent the number.

$\frac{1}{2}n = \frac{2}{3}n-3$

$6(\frac{1}{2}n) = 6(\frac{2}{3}n-3)$

$3n = 4n-18$

$18 = n$

The number is 18.

45. Let n, n+1, and n+2 represent the three consecutive integers.

$n +\frac{1}{3}(n+1) +\frac{3}{8}(n+2) = 25$

$24[n +\frac{1}{3}(n+1) +\frac{3}{8}(n+2)] = 24(25)$

$24n+8(n+1)+9(n+2) = 600$

$24n+8n+8+9n+18 = 600$

$41n+26 = 600$

$41n = 574$

$n = 14$

The integers are 14, 15, and 16.

49. Let n represent Angie's present age. Then 64-n represents her mother's present age. Furthermore, n+8 represents Angie's age in eight years and 64-n+8, which simplifies to 72-n, represents her mother's age in eight years.

$n+8 = \frac{3}{5}(72-n)$

$5(n+8) = 5[\frac{3}{5}(72-n)]$

$5n+40 = 3(72-n)$

$5n+40 = 216-3n$

$8n = 176$

$n = 22$

Angie is 22 years old and her mother is 64-22 = 42 years old.

53. Let x represent the measure of the larger angle. Then $\frac{1}{3}x+4$ represents the measure of the smaller angle. Since they are supplementary angles, the sum of their measures is 180°.

$x + (\frac{1}{3}x+ 4) = 180$

$3[x + (\frac{1}{3}x+ 4)] = 3(180)$

$3x+x+12 = 540$

$4x = 528$

$x = 132$

The measures of the angles are 132° and $\frac{1}{3}(132°) +4° = 48°$.

1.
$$.14x = 2.8$$
$$100(.14x) = 100(2.8)$$
$$14x = 280$$
$$x = 20$$

The solution set is $\{20\}$.

5.
$$n + .4n = 56$$
$$10(n + .4n) = 10(56)$$
$$10n + 4n = 560$$
$$14n = 560$$
$$n = 40$$

The solution set is $\{40\}$.

9.
$$s = 3.3 + .45s$$
$$100(s) = 100(3.3 + .45s)$$
$$100s = 330 + 45s$$
$$55s = 330$$
$$s = 6$$

The solution set is $\{6\}$.

13.
$$.08(x+200) = .07x+20$$
$$100[.08(x+200)] = 100(.07x+20)$$
$$8(x+200) = 7x+2000$$
$$8x+1600 = 7x+2000$$
$$x = 400$$

The solution set is $\{400\}$.

17.
$$.92 + .9(x - .3) = 2x-5.95$$
$$100[.92 + .9(x - .3)] = 100(2x-5.95)$$
$$92+90(x - .3) = 200x-595$$
$$92+90x-27 = 200x-595$$
$$90x+65 = 200x-595$$
$$660 = 110x$$
$$6 = x$$

The solution set is $\{6\}$.

21.
$$.12x + .1(5000-x) = 560$$
$$100[.12x + .1(5000-x)] = 100(560)$$
$$12x+10(5000-x) = 56000$$
$$12x+50000-10x = 56000$$
$$2x = 6000$$
$$x = 3000$$

The solution set is $\{3000\}$.

25.
$$.3(2t + .1) = 8.43$$
$$100[.3(2t + .1)] = 100(8.43)$$
$$30(2t + .1) = 843$$
$$60t+3 = 843$$
$$60t = 840$$
$$t = 14$$

The solution set is $\{14\}$.

29. Let x represent the original price of the coat. Since it was a 20% discount sale, she paid 80% of the original price.

$$.80(x) = 72$$
$$80x = 7200$$
$$x = 90$$

The original price was \$90.

33. Let s represent the selling price. Use the guideline "selling price equals cost plus profit", where the profit is 60% of the cost.

$$s = 30 + .6(30)$$
$$s = 48$$

The selling price should be \$48.

37. Let r represent the rate of profit based on the cost. Use the guideline
     "selling price equals cost plus profit."

$$39.6 = 24 + 24r$$
$$15.6 = 24r$$
$$.65 = r$$

The profit is 65% of the cost.

41. Let x represent the amount invested at 10%. Then x+1500 represents the
     amount invested at 11%.

$$.10x + .11(x+1500) = 795$$
$$10x+11(x+1500) = 79500$$
$$10x+11x+16500 = 79500$$
$$21x = 63000$$
$$x = 3000$$

She invested $3000 at 10% and $3000 + $1500 = $4500 at 11%.

45. Let p represent the number of pennies. Then 2p−1 represents the number of
     nickels and 2p−1+3 = 2p+2 represents the number of dimes. Expressing
     everything in terms of cents, we can solve the following equation.

$$p+5(2p-1)+10(2p+2) = 263$$
$$p+10p-5+20p+20 = 263$$
$$31p+15 = 263$$
$$31p = 248$$
$$p = 8$$

He has 8 pennies, 2(8)−1 = 15 nickels, and 2(8)+2 = 18 dimes.

49.
$$1.2x + 3.4 = 5.2$$
$$10(1.2x + 3.4) = 10(5.2)$$
$$12x+34 = 52$$
$$12x = 18$$
$$x = 1.5$$

The solution set is {1.5}.

53.
$$.7n + 1.4 = 3.92$$
$$100(.7n + 1.4) = 100(3.92)$$
$$70n+140 = 392$$
$$70n = 252$$
$$n = 3.6$$

The solution set is {3.6}.

57.
$$.8(2x-1.4) = 19.52$$
$$100[.8(2x-1.4)] = 100(19.52)$$
$$80(2x-1.4) = 1952$$
$$160x-112 = 1952$$
$$160x = 2064$$
$$x = 12.9$$

The solution set is {12.9}.

Problem Set 2.4

1. $i = Prt$
    $i = 300(.08)(5)$
    $i = 120$

    The interest is $120.

5. $i = Prt$
    $90 = (600)(r)(2.5)$
    $90 = 1500r$
    $.06 = r$

    The rate is 6%.

9. $A = P+Prt$
    $A = 1000+1000(.12)(5)$
    $A = 1000+600$
    $A = 1600$

    The principal is \$1600.

13. $A = P+Prt$
     $326 = P[1+.07(9)]$
     $326 = 1.63P$
     $200 = P$

     The principal is \$200.

17. $V = Bh$

$\frac{1}{B}(V) = \frac{1}{B}(Bh)$ Multiply both sides by $\frac{1}{B}$.

$\frac{V}{B} = h$

21. $C = 2\Pi r$

$\frac{1}{2\Pi}(C) = \frac{1}{2\Pi}(2\Pi r)$ Multiply both sides by $\frac{1}{2\Pi}$.

$\frac{C}{2\Pi} = r$

25. $F = \frac{9}{5}C + 32$

$F-32 = \frac{9}{5}C$ Add -32 to both sides.

$\frac{5}{9}(F-32) = \frac{5}{9}(\frac{9}{5}C)$ Multiply both sides by $\frac{5}{9}$.

$\frac{5}{9}(F-32) = C$

<u>or</u>

$F = \frac{9}{5}C + 32$

$5(F) = 5(\frac{9}{5}C + 32)$ Multiply both sides by 5.

$5F = 9C+160$

$5F-160 = 9C$

$\frac{5F-160}{9} = C$

29. $y-y_1 = m(x-x_1)$

$y-y_1 = mx-mx_1$ Apply distributive property to right side.

$y-y_1+mx_1 = mx$ Add mx_1 to both sides.

$\frac{y-y_1+mx_1}{m} = x$ Multiply both sides by $\frac{1}{m}$.

33. $\frac{x-a}{b} = c$

$x-a = bc$ Multiply both sides by b.

$x = a+bc$ Add <u>a</u> to both sides.

37. $2x-5y = 7$

$2x = 7+5y$ Add 5y to both sides.

$x = \frac{7+5y}{2}$ Multiply both sides by $\frac{1}{2}$.

41. $3(x-2y) = 4$

$3x-6y = 4$ Apply distributive property to left side.

$3x = 4+6y$ Add 6y to both sides.

$x = \dfrac{4+6y}{3}$ Multiply both sides by $\dfrac{1}{3}$.

45. $(y+1)(a-3) = x-2$

$ay-3y+a-3 = x-2$ Find the product on the left side.

$ay-3y = x-2-a+3$ Add $(-a+3)$ to both sides.

$y(a-3) = x-a+1$ Apply distributive property to left side.

$y = \dfrac{x-a+1}{a-3}$ Multiply both sides by $\dfrac{1}{a-3}$.

49. Use the formula $i = Prt$ as a guideline.

$$i = Prt$$
$$500 = 500(.09)t$$
$$1 = .09t$$
$$100 = 9t$$
$$\frac{100}{9} = t$$

It will take $11\frac{1}{9}$ years.

53. A diagram can be used to record the given information and help analyze the problem.

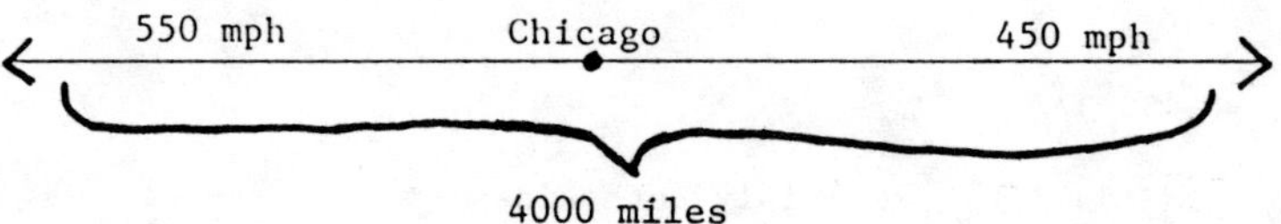

"The distance traveled by one plane plus the distance traveled by the other plane equals 4000 miles" can be used as a guideline. Let t represent the time of each plane since they are the same.

$$550t+450t = 4000$$
$$1000t = 4000$$
$$t = 4$$

At the end of 4 hours they will be 4000 miles apart.

57. This time let's set up a chart to record the given information and help analyze the problem.

	r	t	d
first part of trip	20	x	$20x$
last part of trip	12	$4\frac{1}{2} - x$	$12(4\frac{1}{2}x)$

Notice that we let x represent the time of the first part of the trip and then $4\frac{1}{2} - x$ represents the time of the second part. The formula $d = rt$ is used to fill in the third column. Since the total distance was 70 miles, we can set up and solve the following equation.

$$20x+12(4\tfrac{1}{2} - x) = 70$$
$$20x+54-12x = 70$$
$$8x = 16$$
$$x = 2$$

Bret rode for 2 hours at 20 miles per hour; thus, the first part of the trip was $2(20) = 40$ miles.

61. Let x represent the number of quarts of the 30% solution. Then 20-x
    represents the number of quarts of the 70% solution. Then we can set
    up an equation that represents "pure alcohol in 30% solution plus pure
    alcohol in the 70% solution equals total amount of pure alcohol."

$$.3x + .7(20-x) = .4(20)$$
$$3x+7(20-x) = 4(20)$$
$$3x+140-7x = 80$$
$$-4x = -60$$
$$x = 15$$

We need to mix 15 quarts of the 30% solution with 20-15 = 5 quarts of
the 70% solution.

65.
$$i = Prt$$
$$453.25 = (925)(.14)(t)$$
$$453.25 = 129.5t$$
$$3.5 = t$$

69.
$$A = P+Prt$$
$$1423.50 = P[1+(.095)1]$$
$$1423.50 = 1.095P$$
$$1300 = P$$

Problem Set 2.5

17. $x-3 > -2$
    $x > 1$ Add 3 to both sides.

The solution set is $(1, \infty)$.

21. $5x \le -10$
    $\frac{1}{5}(5x) \le \frac{1}{5}(-10)$ Multiply both sides by $\frac{1}{5}$.
    $x \le -2$

The solution set is $(-\infty, -2]$.

25. $3x-2 > -5$
    $3x > -3$ Add 2 to both sides.
    $\frac{1}{3}(3x) > \frac{1}{3}(-3)$ Multiply both sides by $\frac{1}{3}$.
    $x > -1$

The solution set is $(-1, \infty)$.

29. $2+6x > -10$
    $6x > -12$ Add -2 to both sides.
    $\frac{1}{6}(6x) > \frac{1}{6}(-12)$ Multiply both sides by $\frac{1}{6}$.
    $x > -2$

The solution set is $(-2, \infty)$.

33. $15 < 1-7x$
    $7x+15 < 1$ Add 7x to both sides.
    $7x < -14$ Add -15 to both sides.
    $\frac{1}{7}(7x) < \frac{1}{7}(-14)$ Multiply both sides by $\frac{1}{7}$.
    $x < -2$

The solution set is $(-\infty, -2)$.

37.
$$3(x+2) > 6$$
$$\tfrac{1}{3}[3(x+2)] > \tfrac{1}{3}(6) \qquad \text{Multiply both sides by } \tfrac{1}{3}.$$
$$x+2 > 2$$
$$x > 0 \qquad \text{Add } -2 \text{ to both sides.}$$

The solution set is $(0,\infty)$.

41.
$$2x-1 > 6$$
$$2x > 7 \qquad \text{Add 1 to both sides.}$$
$$\tfrac{1}{2}(2x) > \tfrac{1}{2}(7) \qquad \text{Multiply both sides by } \tfrac{1}{2}.$$
$$x > \tfrac{7}{2}$$

The solution set is $(\tfrac{7}{2},\infty)$.

45.
$$-3(2x+1) \geq 2$$
$$-\tfrac{1}{3}[-3(2x+1)] \leq -\tfrac{1}{3}(12) \qquad \text{Multiply both sides by } -\tfrac{1}{3} \text{ which reverses the inequality.}$$
$$2x+1 \leq -4$$
$$2x \leq -5 \qquad \text{Add } -1 \text{ to both sides.}$$
$$\tfrac{1}{2}(2x) \leq \tfrac{1}{2}(-5) \qquad \text{Multiply both sides by } \tfrac{1}{2}.$$
$$x \leq -\tfrac{5}{2}$$

The solution set is $(-\infty, -\tfrac{5}{2}]$.

49.
$$6x-2 > 4x-14$$
$$2x-2 > -14 \qquad \text{Add } -4x \text{ to both sides.}$$
$$2x > -12 \qquad \text{Add 2 to both sides.}$$
$$\tfrac{1}{2}(2x) > \tfrac{1}{2}(-12) \qquad \text{Multiply both sides by } \tfrac{1}{2}.$$
$$x > -6$$

The solution set is $(-6,\infty)$.

53.
$$4(x-3) \leq -2(x+1)$$
$$4x-12 \leq -2x-2 \qquad \text{Apply distributive property on both sides.}$$
$$6x-12 \leq -2 \qquad \text{Add } 2x \text{ to both sides.}$$
$$6x \leq 10 \qquad \text{Add 12 to both sides.}$$
$$\tfrac{1}{6}(6x) \leq \tfrac{1}{6}(10) \qquad \text{Multiply both sides by } \tfrac{1}{6}.$$
$$x \leq \tfrac{10}{6}$$
$$x \leq \tfrac{5}{3} \qquad \text{Reduce.}$$

The solution set is $(-\infty,\tfrac{5}{3}]$.

57. $\quad -3(3x+2)-2(4x+1) \geq 0$

$\qquad -9x-6-8x-2 \geq 0 \qquad$ Apply distributive property.

$\qquad -17x-8 \geq 0 \qquad$ Combine similar terms.

$\qquad -17x \geq 8 \qquad$ Add 8 to both sides.

$\qquad -\dfrac{1}{17}(-17x) \leq -\dfrac{1}{17}(8) \qquad$ Multiply both sides by $-\dfrac{1}{17}$ which reverses the inequality.

$\qquad x \leq -\dfrac{8}{17}$

The solution set is $\left(-\infty, -\dfrac{8}{17}\right]$.

61. $\quad 7(x+1)-8(x-2) < 0$

$\qquad 7x+7-8x+16 < 0 \qquad$ Apply distributive property.

$\qquad -x+23 < 0 \qquad$ Combine similar terms.

$\qquad -x < -23 \qquad$ Add -23 to both sides.

$\qquad -1(-x) > (-1)(-23) \qquad$ Multiply both sides by -1.

$\qquad x > 23$

The solution set is $(23, \infty)$.

65. $\quad 3(x-2)-5(2x-1) \geq 0$

$\qquad 3x-6-10x+5 \geq 0 \qquad$ Apply distributive property.

$\qquad -7x-1 \geq 0 \qquad$ Combine similar terms.

$\qquad -7x \geq 1 \qquad$ Add 1 to both sides.

$\qquad -\dfrac{1}{7}(-7x) \leq -\dfrac{1}{7} \qquad$ Multiply both sides by $-\dfrac{1}{7}$.

$\qquad x \leq -\dfrac{1}{7}$

The solution set is $\left(-\infty, -\dfrac{1}{7}\right]$.

69. $\quad -3(x+2) > 2(x-6)$

$\qquad -3x-6 > 2x-12 \qquad$ Apply distributive property.

$\qquad -5x-6 > -12 \qquad$ Add $-2x$ to both sides.

$\qquad -5x > -6 \qquad$ Add 6 to both sides.

$\qquad -\dfrac{1}{5}(-5x) < -\dfrac{1}{5}(-6) \qquad$ Multiply both sides by $-\dfrac{1}{5}$.

$\qquad x < \dfrac{6}{5}$

The solution set is $\left(-\infty, \dfrac{6}{5}\right)$.

Problem Set 2.6

1. $\quad \dfrac{2}{5}x + \dfrac{1}{3}x > \dfrac{44}{15}$

$\qquad 15\left(\dfrac{2}{5}x + \dfrac{1}{3}x\right) > 15\left(\dfrac{44}{15}\right)$

$\qquad 6x+5x > 44$

$\qquad 11x > 44$

$\qquad x > 4$

The solution set is $(4, \infty)$.

5. $$\frac{x-2}{3}+\frac{x+1}{4}\geq\frac{5}{2}$$
$$12\left(\frac{x-2}{3}+\frac{x+1}{4}\right)\geq 12\left(\frac{5}{2}\right)$$
$$4(x-2)+3(x+1)\geq 30$$
$$4x-8+3x+3\geq 30$$
$$7x-5\geq 30$$
$$7x\geq 35$$
$$x\geq 5$$

The solution set is $[5,\infty)$.

9. $$\frac{x+3}{8}-\frac{x+5}{5}\geq\frac{3}{10}$$
$$40\left(\frac{x+3}{8}-\frac{x+5}{5}\right)\geq 40\left(\frac{3}{10}\right)$$
$$5(x+3)-8(x+5)\geq 12$$
$$5x+15-8x-40\geq 12$$
$$-3x-25\geq 12$$
$$-3x\geq 37$$
$$-\frac{1}{3}(-3x)\leq -\frac{1}{3}(37)$$
$$x\leq -\frac{37}{3}$$

The solution set is $\left(-\infty, -\frac{37}{3}\right]$.

13. $$.06x+.08(250-x)\geq 19$$
$$100[.06x+.08(250-x)]\geq 100(19)$$
$$6x+8(250-x)\geq 1900$$
$$6x+2000-8x\geq 1900$$
$$-2x\geq -100$$
$$x\leq 50$$

The solution set is $(-\infty,50]$.

17. $$x\geq 3.4+.15x$$
$$100(x)\geq 100(3.4+.15x)$$
$$100x\geq 340+15x$$
$$85x\geq 340$$
$$x\geq 4$$

The solution set is $[4,\infty)$.

21. The "and" means that the solution set is the intersection of all numbers less than or equal to 2 and all numbers greater than -1. Thus, the solution set is $(-1,2]$.

25. The "or" means that the solution set is the union of all numbers less than or equal to 1 along with all numbers greater than 3. Thus, the solution set is $(-\infty,1]\cup(3,\infty)$.

29. There are no numbers that are less than zero and also greater than 4. The solution set is $\emptyset$.

33. The "or" means that the solution set is the union of all numbers greater than -1 along with all numbers greater than 2. Thus, the solution set is $(-1,\infty)$.

37. $$x+2<-3 \text{ or } x+2>3$$
$$x<-5 \text{ or } \quad x>1$$

The solution set is $(-\infty,-5)\cup(1,\infty)$.

41. $$5x-2<0 \text{ and } 3x-1>0$$
$$5x<2 \text{ and } \quad 3x>1$$
$$x<\frac{2}{5} \text{ and } \quad x>\frac{1}{3}$$

The solution set is $\left(\frac{1}{3},\frac{2}{5}\right)$.

45. $$-3<2x+1<5$$
$$-4<2x<4 \qquad \text{Add } -1.$$
$$\frac{1}{2}(-4)<\frac{1}{2}(2x)<\frac{1}{2}(4) \qquad \text{Multiply by } \frac{1}{2}.$$
$$-2<x<2$$

The solution set is $(-2,2)$.

49. $$1<4x+3<9$$
$$-2<4x<6 \qquad \text{Add } -3.$$
$$\frac{1}{4}(-2)<\frac{1}{4}(4x)<\frac{1}{4}(6) \quad \text{Multiply by } \frac{1}{4}.$$
$$-\frac{2}{4}<x<\frac{6}{4}$$
$$-\frac{1}{2}<x<\frac{3}{2}$$

The solution set is $\left(-\frac{1}{2},\frac{3}{2}\right)$.

53. $$-4 \leq \frac{x-1}{3} \leq 4$$

$3(-4) \leq 3(\frac{x-1}{3}) \leq 3(4)$ Multiply by 3.

$-12 \leq x-1 \leq 12$

$-11 \leq x \leq 13$ Add 1.

The solution set is $[-11,13]$.

57. Let r represent the rate of the investment of $200.

$$.09(300)+200r > 47$$
$$27+200r > 47$$
$$200r > 20$$
$$r > \frac{1}{10}$$

It must be invested at a rate greater than 10%.

61. Let x represent her score in the third game.

$$\frac{142+170+x}{3} \geq 160$$
$$142+170+x \geq 480$$
$$312+x \geq 480$$
$$x \geq 168$$

She must get a score of 168 or better.

65. Use the formula $F = \frac{9}{5}C + 32$ and substitute $\frac{9}{5}C + 32$ for F.

$$325 \leq \frac{9}{5}C + 32 \leq 425$$
$$293 \leq \frac{9}{5}C \leq 393$$
$$\frac{5}{9}(293) \leq \frac{5}{9}(\frac{9}{5}C) \leq \frac{5}{9}(393)$$
$$162.\overline{7} \leq C \leq 218.\overline{3}$$

Rounding to the nearest degree we obtain $163 \leq C \leq 218$.

Problem Set 2.7

1. By Property 2.2, $|x| < 5$ is equivalent to $-5 < x < 5$. Thus, the solution set is $(-5,5)$.

5. By Property 2.3, $|x| > 2$ is equivalent to $x < -2$ or $x > 2$. Thus, the solution set is $(-\infty,-2) \cup (2,\infty)$.

9. By Property 2.2, $|x+2| \leq 4$ is equivalent to $-4 \leq x+2 \leq 4$, which can be solved as follows.

$$-4 \leq x+2 \leq 4$$
$$-6 \leq x \leq 2$$

The solution set is $[-6,2]$.

13. By Property 2.3, $|x-3| \geq 2$ is equivalent to $x-3 \leq -2$ or $x-3 \geq 2$, which can be solved as follows.

$$x-3 \leq -2 \text{ or } x-3 \geq 2$$
$$x \leq 1 \quad \text{or} \quad x \geq 5$$

The solution set is $(-\infty,1] \cup [5,\infty)$.

17. By Property 2.3, $|x-2| > 6$ is equivalent to $x-2 < -6$ or $x-2 > 6$, which can be solved as follows.

$$x-2 < -6 \text{ or } x-2 > 6$$
$$x < -4 \text{ or} \quad x > 8$$

The solution set is $(-\infty,-4) \cup (8,\infty)$.

21. By Property 2.1, $|2x-4| = 6$ is equivalent to $2x-4 = -6$ or $2x-4 = 6$, which can be solved as follows.

$$2x-4 = -6 \text{ or } 2x-4 = 6$$
$$2x = -2 \text{ or } 2x = 10$$
$$x = -1 \text{ or } x = 5$$

The solution set is $\{-1,5\}$.

25. By Property 2.3, $|4x+2| \geq 12$ is equivalent to $4x+2 \leq -12$ or $4x+2 \geq 12$, which can be solved as follows.

$$4x+2 \leq -12 \text{ or } 4x+2 \geq 12$$
$$4x \leq -14 \text{ or } 4x \geq 10$$
$$x \leq -\frac{14}{4} \text{ or } x \geq \frac{10}{4}$$
$$x \leq -\frac{7}{2} \text{ or } x \geq \frac{5}{2}$$

The solution set is $(-\infty, -\frac{7}{2}] \cup [\frac{5}{2}, \infty)$.

29. By Property 2.1, $|4-2x| = 6$ is equivalent to $4-2x = -6$ or $4-2x = 6$, which can be solved as follows.

$$4-2x = -6 \text{ or } 4-2x = 6$$
$$-2x = -10 \text{ or } -2x = 2$$
$$x = 5 \text{ or } x = -1$$

The solution set is $\{-1,5\}$.

33. By Property 2.2, $|1-2x| < 2$ is equivalent to $-2 < 1-2x < 2$, which can be solved as follows.

$$-2 < 1-2x < 2$$
$$-3 < -2x < 1$$
$$\frac{3}{2} > x > -\frac{1}{2}$$

The solution set is $(-\frac{1}{2}, \frac{3}{2})$.

37. By Property 2.1, $|x-\frac{3}{4}| = \frac{2}{3}$ is equivalent to $x-\frac{3}{4} = -\frac{2}{3}$ or $x-\frac{3}{4} = \frac{2}{3}$, which can be solved as follows.

$$x-\frac{3}{4} = -\frac{2}{3} \text{ or } x-\frac{3}{4} = \frac{2}{3}$$
$$x = -\frac{2}{3}+\frac{3}{4} \text{ or } x = \frac{2}{3}+\frac{3}{4}$$
$$x = -\frac{8}{12}+\frac{9}{12} \text{ or } x = \frac{8}{12}+\frac{9}{12}$$
$$x = \frac{1}{12} \text{ or } x = \frac{17}{12}$$

The solution set is $\{\frac{1}{12}, \frac{17}{12}\}$.

41. By Property 2.2, $\left|\frac{x-3}{4}\right| < 2$ is equivalent to $-2 < \frac{x-3}{4} < 2$, which can be solved as follows.

$$-2 < \frac{x-3}{4} < 2$$
$$-8 < x-3 < 8$$
$$-5 < x < 11$$

The solution set is $(-5, 11)$.

45. $|2x-3| + 2 = 5$
    $|2x-3| = 3$ Add -2 to both sides.

Now by Property 2.1, $|2x-3| = 3$ is equivalent to $2x-3 = -3$ or $2x-3 = 3$, which can be solved as follows.

$$2x-3 = -3 \text{ or } 2x-3 = 3$$
$$2x = 0 \text{ or } 2x = 6$$
$$x = 0 \text{ or } x = 3$$

The solution set is $\{0, 3\}$.

49. $|2x-1| + 1 \le 6$
    $|2x-1| \le 5$ Add -1 to both sides.

Now by Property 2.2, $|2x-1| \le 5$ is equivalent to $-5 \le 2x-1 \le 5$, which can be solved as follows.

$$-5 \le 2x-1 \le 5$$
$$-4 \le 2x \le 6$$
$$-2 \le x \le 3$$

The solution set is $[-2, 3]$.

53. Because the absolute value of any real number is nonnegative, the solution set for $|3x-1| > -2$ is $(-\infty, \infty)$.

57. Because the absolute value of any real number is nonnegative, the solution set for $|4x-6| < -1$ is $\emptyset$.

Chapter 3

Problem Set 3.1

13. $(-5t-4)+(-6t+9) = [-5+(-6)]t+(-4+9) = -11t+5$

17. $(12a^2b^2-9ab)+(5a^2b^2+4ab) = (12+5)a^2b^2+(-9+4)ab = 17a^2b^2-5ab$

21. $(3x+4)-(5x-2) = 3x+4-5x+2 = -2x+6$

25. $(7x^2+9x+8)-(3x^2-x+2) = 7x^2+9x+8-3x^2+x-2 = 4x^2+10x+6$

29. $(5x^3+2x^2+6x-13)-(2x^3+x^2-7x-2) = 5x^3+2x^2+6x-13-2x^3-x^2+7x+2 = 3x^3+x^2+13x-11$

33. $\begin{array}{l} -7x-9 \\ \underline{-4x+7} \\ -3x-16 \end{array}$ ⟵ Form the opposite of this polynomial and add.

37. $\begin{array}{l} -2x^3+6x^2-3x+8 \\ \underline{x^3+x^2-x-1} \\ -3x^3+5x^2-2x+9 \end{array}$ ⟵ Form the opposite of this polynomial and add.

41. $(x^2+9x-4)+(-5x^2-7x+10)-(2x^2-7x-1) = x^2+9x-4-5x^2-7x+10-2x^2+7x+1 = -6x^2+9x+7$

45. $(-12n^2-n+9)-[(5n^2-3n-2)+(-7n^2+n+2)] = (-12n^2-n+9)-(-2n^2-2n)$
$$= -12n^2-n+9+2n^2+2n = -10n^2+n+9$$

49. $(12x-9)-(-3x+4)-(7x+1) = 12x-9+3x-4-7x-1 = 8x-14$

53. $(7x^2-x-4)-(9x^2-10x+8)+(12x^2+4x-6) = 7x^2-x-4-9x^2+10x-8+12x^2+4x-6$
$$= 10x^2+13x-18$$

57. $3x-[5x-(x+6)] = 3x-[5x-x-6] = 3x-[4x-6] = 3x-4x+6 = -x+6$

61. $-2n^2-[n^2-(-4n^2+n+6)] = -2n^2-[n^2+4n^2-n-6] = -2n^2-[5n^2-n-6]$
$$= -2n^2-5n^2+n+6 = -7n^2+n+6$$

65. $[2n^2-(2n^2-n+5)]+[3n^2+(n^2-2n-7)] = [2n^2-2n^2+n-5]+[3n^2+n^2-2n-7]$
$$= [n-5]+[4n^2-2n-7] = 4n^2-n-12$$

69. $[4x^3-(2x^2-x-1)]-[5x^3-(x^2+2x-1)] = [4x^3-2x^2+x+1]-[5x^3-x^2-2x+1]$
$$= 4x^3-2x^2+x+1-5x^3+x^2+2x-1 = -x^3-x^2+3x$$

Problem Set 3.2

1. $(4x^3)(9x) = 36x^{3+1} = 36x^4$

5. $(-a^2b)(-4ab^3) = 4a^{2+1}b^{1+3} = 4a^3b^4$

9. $(5xy)(-6y^3) = -30xy^{1+3} = -30xy^4$

13. $(m^2n)(-mn^2) = -m^{2+1}n^{1+2} = -m^3n^3$

17. $(-\frac{3}{4}ab)(\frac{1}{5}a^2b^3) = (-\frac{3}{4})(\frac{1}{5})a^{1+2}b^{1+3} = -\frac{3}{20}a^3b^4$

21. $(3x)(-2x^2)(-5x^3) = 30x^{1+2+3} = 30x^6$

25. $(x^2y)(-3xy^2)(x^3y^3) = -3x^{2+1+3}y^{1+2+3} = -3x^6y^6$

29. $(4ab)(-2a^2b)(7a) = -56a^{1+2+1}b^{1+1} = -56a^4b^2$

33. $(\frac{2}{3}xy)(-3x^2y)(5x^4y^5) = -10x^{1+2+4}y^{1+1+5} = -10x^7y^7$

37. $(3xy^2)^3 = (3)^3(x)^3(y^2)^3 = 27x^3y^6$ 41. $(-x^4y^5)^4 = (-1)^4(x^4)^4(y^5)^4 = x^{16}y^{20}$

45. $(2a^2b^3)^6 = (2)^6(a^2)^6(b^3)^6 = 64a^{12}b^{18}$

49. $(-3ab^3)^4 = (-3)^4(a^4)(b^3)^4 = 81a^4b^{12}$

53. $-(xy^2z^3)^6 = [(x)^6(y^2)^6(z^3)^6] = -x^6y^{12}z^{18}$

57. $(-xy^4z^2)^7 = (-1)^7(x)^7(y^4)^7(z^2)^7 = -x^7y^{28}z^{14}$

61. $\dfrac{25x^5y^6}{-5x^2y^4} = -5x^{5-2}y^{6-4} = -5x^3y^2$

65. $\dfrac{-18x^2y^2z^6}{xyz^2} = -18x^{2-1}y^{2-1}z^{6-2} = -18xyz^4$

69. $\dfrac{-72x^2y^4}{-8x^2y^4} = 9(1)(1) = 9$ 73. $\dfrac{-36x^3y^5}{2y^5} = -18x^3(1) = -18x^3$

77. $(a^{2n-1})(a^{3n+4}) = a^{2n-1+3n+4} = a^{5n+3}$ 81. $(a^{5n-2})(a^3) = a^{5n-2+3} = a^{5n+1}$

85. $(-3a^2)(-4a^{n+2}) = 12a^{2+n+2} = 12a^{n+4}$

89. $(3x^{n-1})(x^{n+1})(4x^{2-n}) = 12x^{n-1+n+1+2-n} = 12x^{n+2}$

Problem Set 3.3

1. $2xy(5xy^2+3x^2y^3) = 2xy(5xy^2)+2xy(3x^2y^3) = 10x^2y^3+6x^3y^4$

5. $8a^3b^4(3ab-2ab^2+4a^2b^2) = 8a^3b^4(3ab)-8a^3b^4(2ab^2)+8a^3b^4(4a^2b^2)$
$$= 24a^4b^5-16a^4b^6+32a^5b^6$$

9. $(a+2b)(x+y) = a(x+y)+2b(x+y) = ax+ay+2bx+2by$

13. $(x+6)(x+10) = x(x+10)+6(x+10) = x^2+10x+6x+60 = x^2+16x+60$

17. $(n+2)(n-7) = n(n-7)+2(n-7) = n^2-7n+2n-14 = n^2-5n-14$

21. Apply the pattern $(a-b)^2 = a^2-2ab+b^2$.

    $(x-6)^2 = x^2-2(x)(6)+6^2 = x^2-12x+36$

25. $(x+1)(x-2)(x-3) = (x+1)(x^2-5x+6) = x(x^2-5x+6)+1(x^2-5x+6)$
$$= x^3-5x^2+6x+x^2-5x+6 = x^3-4x^2+x+6$$

29. Apply the pattern $(a+b)^2 = a^2+2ab+b^2$.

    $(t+9)^2 = t^2+2(t)(9)+9^2 = t^2+18t+81$

33. $(4x+5)(x+7) = 4x(x+7)+5(x+7) = 4x^2+28x+5x+35 = 4x^2+33x+35$

37. $(7x-2)(2x+1) = 7x(2x+1)-2(2x+1) = 14x^2+7x-4x-2 = 14x^2+3x-2$

41. Use the pattern $(a+b)^2 = a^2+2ab+b^2$.

$$(3t+7)^2 = (3t)^2+2(3t)(7)+7^2$$
$$= 9t^2+42t+49$$

45. Use the pattern $(a-b)^2 = a^2-2ab+b^2$.

$$(7x-4)^2 = (7x)^2-2(7x)(4)+4^2 = 49x^2-56x+16$$

49. $(2x-5y)(x+3y) = 2x(x+3y)-5y(x+3y) = 2x^2+6xy-5xy-15y^2 = 2x^2+xy-15y^2$

53. $(t+3)(t^2-3t-5) = t(t^2-3t-5)+3(t^2-3t-5) = t^3-3t^2-5t+3t^2-9t-15 = t^3-14t-15$

57. $(2x-3)(x^2+6x+10) = 2x(x^2+6x+10)-3(x^2+6x+10) = 2x^3+12x^2+20x-3x^2-18x-30$
$$= 2x^3+9x^2+2x-30$$

61. $(x^2+2x+1)(x^2+3x+4) = x^2(x^2+3x+4)+2x(x^2+3x+4)+1(x^2+3x+4)$
$$= x^4+3x^3+4x^2+2x^3+6x^2+8x+x^2+3x+4 = x^4+5x^3+11x^2+11x+4$$

65. $(x+2)^3 = x^3+3x^2(2)+3x(2)^2+2^3 = x^3+6x^2+12x+8$

69. $(2x+3)^3 = (2x)^3+3(2x)^2(3)+3(2x)(3)^2+3^3 = 8x^3+36x^2+54x+27$

73. $(5x+2)^3 = (5x)^3+3(5x)^2(2)+3(5x)(2)^2+2^3 = 125x^3+150x^2+60x+8$

77. $(x^a+6)(x^a-2) = x^a(x^a-2)+6(x^a-2) = x^{2a}-2x^a+6x^a-12 = x^{2a}+4x^a-12$

81. $(x^{2a}-7)(x^{2a}-3) = x^{2a}(x^{2a}-3)-7(x^{2a}-3) = x^{4a}-3x^{2a}-7x^{2a}+21 = x^{4a}-10x^{2a}+21$

Problem Set 3.4

1. $63 = 9 \cdot 7$; thus, 63 is a composite number.

5. $51 = 3 \cdot 17$; thus, 51 is a composite number.

9. 71 is a prime number because it has no divisors other than 1 and itself.

13. $44 = 4 \cdot 11 = 2 \cdot 2 \cdot 11$ 17. $72 = 8 \cdot 9 = 2 \cdot 2 \cdot 2 \cdot 3 \cdot 3$

21. $6x+3y = 3(2x)+3(y) = 3(2x+y)$ 25. $28y^2-4y = 4y(7y)-4y(1) = 4y(7y-1)$

29. $7x^3+10x^2 = x^2(7x)+x^2(10) = x^2(7x+10)$

33. $12x^3y^4-39x^4y^3 = 3x^3y^3(4y)-3x^3y^3(13x) = 3x^3y^3(4y-13x)$

37. $5x+7x^2+9x^4 = x(5)+x(7x)+x(9x^3) = x(5+7x+9x^3)$

41. $x(y+2)+3(y+2) = (y+2)(x+3)$ 45. $x(x+2)+5(x+2) = (x+2)(x+5)$

49. $ax-2bx+ay-2by = x(a-2b)+y(a-2b) = (a-2b)(x+y)$

53. $2ax+2x+ay+y = 2x(a+1)+y(a+1) = (a+1)(2x+y)$

57. $2ac+3bd+2bc+3ad = 2ac+2bc+3bd+3ad = 2c(a+b)+3d(b+a)$
$$= 2c(a+b)+3d(a+b) = (a+b)(2c+3d)$$

61. $x^2+9x+6x+54 = x(x+9)+6(x+9) = (x+9)(x+6)$

65. $x^2+7x = 0$

          $x(x+7) = 0$ Factor left side.

    $x = 0$ or $x+7 = 0$ Apply Property 3.5.

    $x = 0$ or $x = -7$

The solution set is $\{-7,0\}$.

69. $a^2 = 5a$

     $a^2-5a = 0$ Add $-5a$ to both sides.

     $a(a-5) = 0$ Factor left side.

  $a = 0$ or $a-5 = 0$ Apply Property 3.5.

  $a = 0$ or $a = 5$

The solution set is $\{0,5\}$.

73. $3x^2+7x = 0$

       $x(3x+7) = 0$ Factor left side.

   $x = 0$ or $3x+7 = 0$ Apply Property 3.5.

   $x = 0$ or $3x = -7$

   $x = 0$ or $x = -\dfrac{7}{3}$

The solution set is $\{-\frac{7}{3}, 0\}$.

77. $x-4x^2 = 0$

      $x(1-4x) = 0$ Factor left side.

  $x = 0$ or $1-4x = 0$ Apply Property 3.5.

  $x = 0$ or $-4x = -1$

  $x = 0$ or $x = \dfrac{1}{4}$

The solution set is $\{0,\frac{1}{4}\}$.

81. $5bx^2-3ax = 0$

       $x(5bx-3a) = 0$ Factor left side.

  $x = 0$ or $5bx-3a = 0$ Apply Property 3.5.

  $x = 0$ or $5bx = 3a$

  $x = 0$ or $x = \dfrac{3a}{5b}$

The solution set is $\{0,\frac{3a}{5b}\}$.

85. $y^2-ay+2by-2ab = 0$

    $y(y-a)+2b(y-a) = 0$

      $(y-a)(y+2b) = 0$

   $y-a = 0$ or $y+2b = 0$

    $y = a$ or $y = -2b$

The solution set is $\{a,-2b\}$.

89. Let r represent the length of a radius.

      $\pi r^2 = 3(2\pi r)$

      $\pi r^2 = 6\pi r$

   $\pi r^2-6\pi r = 0$

    $\pi r(r-6) = 0$

  $\pi r = 0$ or $r-6 = 0$

   $r = 0$ or $r = 6$

The length of a radius is 6 units.

93.

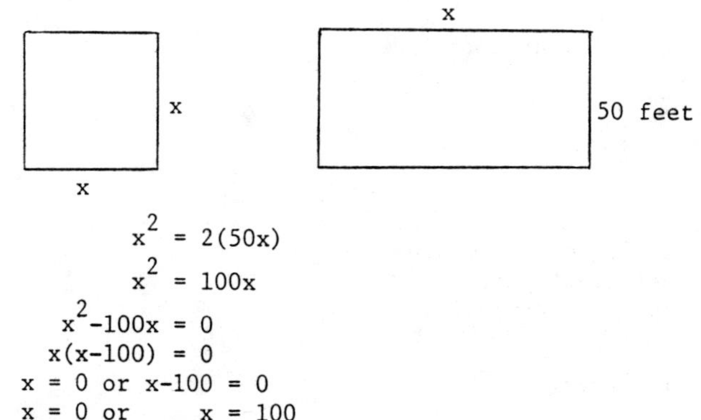

$$x^2 = 2(50x)$$
$$x^2 = 100x$$
$$x^2-100x = 0$$
$$x(x-100) = 0$$
$$x = 0 \text{ or } x-100 = 0$$
$$x = 0 \text{ or } x = 100$$

The square is 100 feet by 100 feet and the rectangle is 50 feet by 100 feet.

Problem Set 3.5

1. $x^2-1 = x^2-1^2 = (x+1)(x-1)$

5. $9x^2-25y^2 = (3x)^2-(5y)^2 = (3x+5y)(3x-5y)$

9. $4x^2-y^4 = (2x)^2-(y^2)^2 = (2x+y^2)(2x-y^2)$

13. $(x+2)^2-y^2 = (x+2+y)(x+2-y)$

17. $9a^2-(2b+3)^2 = (3a)^2-(2b+3)^2 = [3a+(2b-3)][3a-(2b+3)] = (3a+2b+3)(3a-2b-3)$

21. $9x^2-36 = 9(x^2-4) = 9(x+2)(x-2)$ 25. $8y^2-32 = 8(y^2-4) = 8(y+2)(y-2)$

29. There is no common factor and the sum of two squares is not factorable.

33. $3x^3+27x = 3x(x^2+9)$ 37. $6x-6x^3 = 6x(1-x^2) = 6x(1+x)(1-x)$

41. $4x^2-64y^2 = 4(x^2-16y^2) = 4(x+4y)(x-4y)$ 45. $a^3-64 = (a-4)(a^2+4a+16)$

49. $27x^3+64y^3 = (3x+4y)(9x^2-12xy+16y^2)$ 53. $x^3y^3-1 = (xy-1)(x^2y^2+xy+1)$

57. $$x^2-25 = 0$$
$$(x+5)(x-5) = 0$$
$$x+5 = 0 \text{ or } x-5 = 0$$
$$x = -5 \text{ or } x = 5$$

The solution set is $\{-5,5\}$.

61. $$8x^2-32 = 0$$
$$\tfrac{1}{8}(8x^2-32) = \tfrac{1}{8}(0)$$
$$x^2-4 = 0$$
$$(x+2((x-2) = 0$$
$$x+2 = 0 \text{ or } x-2 = 0$$
$$x = -2 \text{ or } x = 2$$

The solution set is $\{-2,2\}$.

65.

$$20-5x^2 = 0$$
$$\tfrac{1}{5}(20-5x^2) = \tfrac{1}{5}(0)$$
$$4-x^2 = 0$$
$$(2+x)(2-x) = 0$$
$$2+x = 0 \quad \text{or} \quad 2-x = 0$$
$$x = -2 \quad \text{or} \quad 2 = x$$

The solution set is $\{-2,2\}$.

69.

$$6x^3+24x = 0$$
$$6x(x^2+4) = 0$$
$$6x = 0 \text{ or } x^2+4 = 0$$
$$x = 0 \text{ or } \quad x^2 = -4$$

The equation $x^2 = -4$ has no real number solutions. Thus, the solution set of the given equation is $\{0\}$.

73. Let r represent the length of a radius of the smaller circle. Then 2r represents the length of a radius of the larger circle.

$$\pi r^2+\pi(2r)^2 = 80\pi$$
$$\pi r^2+4\pi r^2 = 80\pi$$
$$5\pi r^2 = 80\pi$$
$$\tfrac{1}{5\pi}(5\pi r^2) = \tfrac{1}{5\pi}(80\pi)$$
$$r^2 = 16$$
$$r^2-16 = 0$$
$$(r+4)(r-4) = 0$$
$$r+4 = 0 \text{ or } r-4 = 0$$
$$r = -4 \text{ or } \quad r = 4$$

Disregarding the negative answer, the length of a radius of the smaller circle is 4 centimeters and of the larger circle is 2(4) = 8 centimeters.

77. Let r represent the length of a radius. Then 2r represents the length of the altitude.

$$2\pi r^2+2\pi r(2r) = 54\pi$$
$$2\pi r^2+4\pi r^2 = 54\pi$$
$$6\pi r^2 = 54\pi$$
$$r^2 = 9$$
$$r^2-9 = 0$$
$$(r+3)(r-3) = 0$$
$$r+3 = 0 \text{ or } r-3 = 0$$
$$r = -3 \text{ or } \quad r = 3$$

The altitude is 2(3) = 6 inches.

Problem Set 3.6

1. We need two integers whose sum is 9 and whose product is 20. They are 4 and 5.
$$x^2+9x+20 = (x+4)(x+5)$$

5. We need two integers whose sum is 5 and whose product is -36. They are 9 and -4.
$$a^2+5a-36 = (a+9)(a-4)$$

9. We need two integers whose sum is -5 and whose product is -14. They are -7 and 2.
$$x^2-5x-14 = (x-7)(x+2)$$

13. $6+5x-x^2 = (6-x)(1+x)$

17.   We need two integers whose sum is −1 and whose product is −56. They are −8 and 7.

$$a^2-ab-56b^2 = (a-8b)(a+7b)$$

21. $12x^2-x-6$ ⟶ sum of −1

product of $12(-6) = -72$

We need two integers whose sum is −1 and whose product is −72. They are −9 and 8.

$$12x^2-x-6 = 12x^2-9x+8x-6 = 3x(4x-3)+2(4x-3) = (4x-3)(3x+2)$$

25. $12n^2-43n-20$ ⟶ sum of −43

product of $12(-20) = -240$

We need two integers whose sum is −43 and whose product is −240. They are −48 and 5.

$$12n^2-43n-20 = 12n^2-48n+5n-20 = 12n(n-4)+5(n-4) = (n-4)(12n+5)$$

29. $20n^2-64n-21$ ⟶ sum of −64

product of $20(-21) = -420$

We need two integers whose sum is −64 and whose product is −420. They are −70 and 6.

$$20n^2-64n-21 = 20n^2-70n+6n-21 = 10n(2n-7)+3(2n-7) = (2n-7)(10n+3)$$

33. $6-29x-42x^2 = -42x^2-29x+6 = -(42x^2+29x-6)$

To factor $42x^2+29x-6$ we need two integers whose sum is 29 and whose product is $42(-6) = -252$. They are 36 and −7.

$$-(42x^2+29x-6) = -[42x^2+36x-7x-6] = -[6x(7x+6)-1(7x+6)]$$
$$= -[7x+6)(6x-1)] = (1-6x)(6+7x)$$

37. $24n^2-2n-5$ ⟶ sum of −2

product of $24(-5) = -120$

We need two integers whose sum is −2 and whose product is −120. They are −12 and 10.

$$24n^2-2n-5 = 24n^2-12n+10n-5 = 12n(2n-1)+5(2n-1) = (2n-1)(12n+5)$$

41. We need two integers whose sum is 25 and whose product is 150. They are
     10 and 15.
$$x^2+25x+150 = (x+10)(x+15)$$

45. We need two integers whose sum is 3 and whose product is −180. They are
     15 and −12.
$$t^2+3t-180 = (t+15)(t-12)$$

49. $10x^4+3x^2-4 = (2x^2-1)(5x^2+4)$

53. $18n^4+25n^2-3 = (9n^2-1)(2n^2+3) = (3n+1)(3n-1)(2n^2+3)$

57. $2t^2-8 = 2(t^2-4) = 2(t+2)(t-2)$

61. $18n^3+39n^2-15n = 3n(6n^2+13n-5) = 3n(2n+5)(3n-1)$

65. $36a^2-12a+1 = (6a-1)(6a-1) = (6a-1)^2$

69. $3x^2+x-5$ $\longrightarrow$ sum of 1

     product of $3(-5) = -15$

     We need two integers whose sum is 1 and whose product is −15. There are
     no two integers that satisfy these conditions; thus, the given polynomial
     is not factorable.

73. $1-16x^4 = (1-4x^2)(1+4x^2) = (1+2x)(1-2x)(1+4x^2)$

77. $n^3-49n = n(n^2-49) = n(n+7)(n-7)$

81. $3x^4-81x = 3x(x^3-27) = 3x(x-3)(x^2+3x+9)$

85. $x^4-5x^2-36 = (x^2-9)(x^2+4) = (x+3)(x-3)(x^2+4)$

89. There is no common factor and the sum of two squares is not factorable.
     Thus, the given polynomial is not factorable.

93. $2xy+6x+y+3 = 2x(y+3)+1(y+3) = (y+3)(2x+1)$

Problem Set 3.7

1. $x^2+4x+3 = 0$
      $(x+3)(x+1) = 0$
      $x+3 = 0$ or $x+1 = 0$
      $x = -3$ or $x = -1$

      The solution set is $\{-3,-1\}$.

5. $n^2-13n+36 = 0$
      $(n-4)(n-9) = 0$
      $n-4 = 0$ or $n-9 = 0$
      $n = 4$ or $n = 9$

      The solution set is $\{4,9\}$.

9. $w^2-4w = 5$
      $w^2-4w-5 = 0$
      $(w-5)(w+1) = 0$
      $w-5 = 0$ or $w+1 = 0$
      $w = 5$ or $w = -1$

      The solution set is $\{-1,5\}$.

13. $3t^2+14t-5 = 0$
      $(3t-1)(t+5) = 0$
      $3t-1 = 0$ or $t+5 = 0$
      $3t = 1$ or $t = -5$
      $t = \dfrac{1}{3}$ or $t = -5$

      The solution set is $\{-5,\dfrac{1}{3}\}$.

17. $$3t(t-4) = 0$$
$$3t = 0 \text{ or } t-4 = 0$$
$$t = 0 \text{ or } t = 4$$

The solution set is $\{0,4\}$.

21. $$2n^3 = 72n$$
$$n^3 = 36n$$
$$n^3 - 36n = 0$$
$$n(n^2 - 36) = 0$$
$$n(n+6)(n-6) = 0$$
$$n = 0 \text{ or } n+6 = 0 \text{ or } n-6 = 0$$
$$n = 0 \text{ or } n = -6 \text{ or } n = 6$$

The solution set is $\{-6,0,6\}$.

25. $$16 - x^4 = 0$$
$$(4-x^2)(4+x^2) = 0$$
$$(2-x)(2+x)(4+x^2) = 0$$
$$2-x = 0 \text{ or } 2+x = 0 \text{ or } 4+x^2 = 0$$
$$2 = x \text{ or } x = -2 \text{ or } x^2 = -4$$

The equation $x^2 = -4$ has no real number solutions. Therefore, the solution set of the given equation is $\{-2,2\}$.

29. $$3x^2 = 75$$
$$x^2 = 25$$
$$x^2 - 25 = 0$$
$$(x+5)(x-5) = 0$$
$$x+5 = 0 \text{ or } x-5 = 0$$
$$x = -5 \text{ or } x = 5$$

The solution set is $\{-5,5\}$.

33. $$8n^2 - 47n - 6 = 0$$
$$(8n+1)(n-6) = 0$$
$$8n+1 = 0 \text{ or } n-6 = 0$$
$$8n = -1 \text{ or } n = 6$$
$$n = -\frac{1}{8} \text{ or } n = 6$$

The solution set is $\{-\frac{1}{8}, 6\}$.

37. $$35n^2 - 18n - 8 = 0$$
$$(7n+2)(5n-4) = 0$$
$$7n+2 = 0 \text{ or } 5n-4 = 0$$
$$7n = -2 \text{ or } 5n = 4$$
$$n = -\frac{2}{7} \text{ or } n = \frac{4}{5}$$

The solution set is $\{-\frac{2}{7}, \frac{4}{5}\}$.

41. $$n(n+2) = 360$$
$$n^2 + 2n - 360 = 0$$
$$(n+20)(n-18) = 0$$
$$n+20 = 0 \text{ or } n-18 = 0$$
$$n = -20 \text{ or } n = 18$$

The solution set is $\{-20,18\}$.

45. $$3x^4 - 46x^2 - 32 = 0$$
$$(3x^2+2)(x^2-16) = 0$$
$$(3x^2+2)(x+4)(x-4) = 0$$
$$3x^2+2 = 0 \text{ or } x+4 = 0 \text{ or } x-4 = 0$$
$$3x^2 = -2 \text{ or } x = -4 \text{ or } x = 4$$

The equation $3x^2 = -2$ has no real number solutions. Therefore, the solution set of the given equation is $\{-4,4\}$.

49. $$12x^3+46x^2+40x = 0$$
$$2x(6x^2+23x+20) = 0$$
$$2x(2x+5)(3x+4) = 0$$
$$2x = 0 \text{ or } 2x+5 = 0 \text{ or } 3x+4 = 0$$
$$x = 0 \text{ or } 2x = -5 \text{ or } 3x = -4$$
$$x = 0 \text{ or } x = -\frac{5}{2} \text{ or } x = -\frac{4}{3}$$

The solution set is $\{-\frac{5}{2}, -\frac{4}{3}, 0\}$.

53. $$4a(a+1) = 3$$
$$4a^2+4a-3 = 0$$
$$(2a-1)(2a+3) = 0$$
$$2a-1 = 0 \text{ or } 2a+3 = 0$$
$$2a = 1 \text{ or } 2a = -3$$
$$a = \frac{1}{2} \text{ or } a = -\frac{3}{2}$$

The solution set is $\{-\frac{3}{2}, \frac{1}{2}\}$.

57. Let n represent one integer and then 2n+1 represents the other.

$$n(2n+1) = 105$$
$$2n^2+n-105 = 0$$
$$(2n+15)(n-7) = 0$$
$$2n+15 = 0 \text{ or } n-7 = 0$$
$$2n = -15 \text{ or } n = 7$$
$$n = -\frac{15}{2} \text{ or } n = 7$$

Since we are looking for integers, the solution $-\frac{15}{2}$ has to be discarded. Thus, the integers are 7 and 2(7)+1 = 15.

61. Let n and n+1 represent the two consecutive integers.

$$n^2+(n+1)^2 = 85$$
$$n^2+n^2+2n+1 = 85$$
$$2n^2+2n-84 = 0$$
$$n^2+n-42 = 0$$
$$(n+7)(n-6) = 0$$
$$n+7 = 0 \text{ or } n-6 = 0$$
$$n = -7 \text{ or } n = 6$$

The integers are -7 and -7+1 = 6 or 6 and 6+1 = 7.

65. Let n, n+1, and n+2 represent the lengths of the three sides.

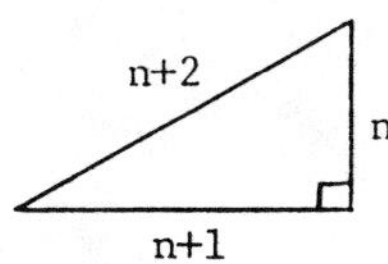

Use the Pythagorean Theorem as a guideline.

$$n^2+(n+1)^2 = (n+2)^2$$
$$n^2+n^2+2n+1 = n^2+4n+4$$
$$2n^2+2n+1 = n^2+4n+4$$
$$n^2-2n-3 = 0$$
$$(n-3)(n+1) = 0$$
$$n-3 = 0 \text{ or } n+1 = 0$$
$$n = 3 \text{ or } n = -1$$

The negative answer must be discarded since we are working with lengths of sides of a triangle. Thus, the sides are of length 3, 4, and 5 units.

69.

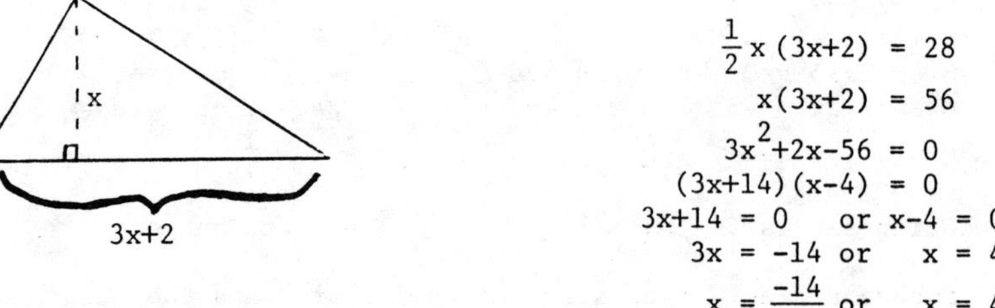

$$\frac{1}{2}x(3x+2) = 28$$
$$x(3x+2) = 56$$
$$3x^2+2x-56 = 0$$
$$(3x+14)(x-4) = 0$$
$$3x+14 = 0 \quad \text{or} \quad x-4 = 0$$
$$3x = -14 \quad \text{or} \quad x = 4$$
$$x = \frac{-14}{3} \quad \text{or} \quad x = 4$$

Again we must discard the negative solution. Thus, the altitude is
4 inches and the length of the side is 3(4)+2 = 14 inches.

Chapter 4

Problem Set 4.1

1. $\dfrac{27}{36} = \dfrac{9 \cdot 3}{9 \cdot 4} = \dfrac{3}{4}$

5. $\dfrac{24}{-60} = -\dfrac{24}{60} = -\dfrac{12 \cdot 2}{12 \cdot 5} = -\dfrac{2}{5}$

9. $\dfrac{12xy}{42y} = \dfrac{2 \cdot 2 \cdot 3 \cdot x \cdot y}{2 \cdot 3 \cdot 7 \cdot y} = \dfrac{2x}{7}$

13. $\dfrac{-14y^3}{56xy^2} = -\dfrac{2 \cdot 7 \cdot y \cdot y \cdot y}{2 \cdot 2 \cdot 2 \cdot 7 \cdot x \cdot y \cdot y} = -\dfrac{y}{4x}$

17. $\dfrac{-40x^3y}{-24xy^4} = \dfrac{2 \cdot 2 \cdot 2 \cdot 5 \cdot x \cdot x \cdot x \cdot y}{2 \cdot 2 \cdot 2 \cdot 3 \cdot x \cdot y \cdot y \cdot y \cdot y} = \dfrac{5x^2}{3y^3}$

21. $\dfrac{18x+12}{12x-6} = \dfrac{6(3x+2)}{6(2x-1)} = \dfrac{3x+2}{2x-1}$

25. $\dfrac{2n^2+n-21}{10n^2+33n-7} = \dfrac{(2n+7)(n-3)}{(2n+7)(5n-1)} = \dfrac{n-3}{5n-1}$

29. $\dfrac{6x^2+x-15}{8x^2-10x-3} = \dfrac{(2x-3)(3x+5)}{(2x-3)(4x+1)} = \dfrac{3x+5}{4x+1}$

33. $\dfrac{3x^2+17x-6}{9x^2-6x+1} = \dfrac{(3x-1)(x+6)}{(3x-1)(3x-1)} = \dfrac{x+6}{3x-1}$

37. $\dfrac{5y^2+22y+8}{25y^2-4} = \dfrac{(5y+2)(y+4)}{(5y+2)(5y-2)} = \dfrac{y+4}{5y-2}$

41. $\dfrac{4x^2y+8xy^2-12y^3}{18x^3y-12x^2y^2-6xy^3} = \dfrac{4y(x^2+2xy-3y^2)}{6xy(3x^2-2xy-y^2)} = \dfrac{4y(x-y)(x+3y)}{6xy(3x+y)(x-y)} = \dfrac{2(x+3y)}{3x(3x+y)}$

45. $\dfrac{8+18x-5x^2}{10+31x+15x^2} = \dfrac{(4-x)(2+5x)}{(5+3x)(2+5x)} = \dfrac{4-x}{5+3x}$

49. $\dfrac{-40x^3+24x^2+16x}{20x^3+28x^2+8x} = \dfrac{-8x(5x^2-3x-2)}{4x(5x^2+7x+2)} = -\dfrac{8x(5x+2)(x-1)}{4x(5x+2)(x+1)} = -\dfrac{2(x-1)}{x+1}$

53. $\dfrac{ax-3x+2ay-6y}{2ax-6x+ay-3y} = \dfrac{x(a-3)-2y(a-3)}{2x(a-3)+y(a-3)} = \dfrac{(a-3)(x-2y)}{(a-3)(2x+y)} = \dfrac{x-2y}{2x+y}$

57. $\dfrac{2st-30-12s+5t}{3st-6-18s+t} = \dfrac{2st-12s+5t-30}{3st-18s+t-6} = \dfrac{2s(t-6)+5(t-6)}{3s(t-6)+1(t-6)} = \dfrac{(t-6)(2s+5)}{(t-6)(3s+1)} = \dfrac{2s+5}{3s+1}$

61. $\dfrac{n^2-49}{7-n} = \dfrac{(n-7)(n+7)}{7-n} = \left(\dfrac{n-7}{7-n}\right)(n+7) = -1(n+7) = -n-7$

65. $\dfrac{2x^3-8x}{4x-x^3} = \dfrac{2x(x^2-4)}{x(4-x^2)} = \left(\dfrac{2x}{x}\right)\left(\dfrac{x^2-4}{4-x^2}\right) = 2(-1) = -2$

Problem Set 4.2

1. $\dfrac{7}{12} \cdot \dfrac{6}{35} = \dfrac{7 \cdot 6}{12 \cdot 35} = \dfrac{1}{10}$

5. $\dfrac{3}{-8} \cdot \dfrac{-6}{12} = \left(-\dfrac{3}{8}\right)\left(-\dfrac{6}{12}\right) = \dfrac{3 \cdot 6}{8 \cdot 12} = \dfrac{3}{16}$

9. $\dfrac{-9}{5} \div \dfrac{27}{10} = \left(-\dfrac{9}{5}\right)\left(\dfrac{10}{27}\right) = -\dfrac{9 \cdot 10}{5 \cdot 27} = -\dfrac{2}{3}$

13. $\dfrac{6xy}{9y^4} \cdot \dfrac{30x^3y}{-48x} = -\dfrac{\cancel{6} \cdot \overset{\overset{5}{\cancel{10}}}{\cancel{30}} \cdot \overset{x^3}{\cancel{x^4}} \cdot \cancel{y^2}}{\underset{\underset{4}{\cancel{8}}}{\cancel{9}} \cdot \cancel{48} \cdot \cancel{x} \cdot \underset{y^2}{\cancel{y^4}}} = -\dfrac{5x^3}{12y^2}$

17. $\dfrac{5xy}{8y^2} \cdot \dfrac{18x^2y}{15} = \dfrac{\cancel{5} \cdot \overset{3}{\cancel{18}} \cdot x^3 \cdot \cancel{y^2}}{\underset{4}{\cancel{8}} \cdot \underset{3}{\cancel{15}} \cdot \cancel{y^2}} = \dfrac{3x^3}{4}$

21. $\dfrac{9a^2c}{12bc^2} \div \dfrac{21ab}{14c^3} = \dfrac{9a^2c}{12bc^2} \cdot \dfrac{14c^3}{21ab} = \dfrac{\overset{3}{\cancel{9}} \cdot \overset{\cancel{7}}{\cancel{14}} \cdot \overset{a}{\cancel{a^2}} \cdot \overset{c^2}{\cancel{c^4}}}{\underset{\underset{2}{\cancel{6}}}{\cancel{12}} \cdot \underset{\cancel{7}}{\cancel{21}} \cdot \cancel{a} \cdot b^2 \cdot \cancel{c^3}} = \dfrac{ac^2}{2b^2}$

25. $\dfrac{3x+6}{5y} \cdot \dfrac{x^2+4}{x^2+10x+16} = \dfrac{3\cancel{(x+2)}(x^2+4)}{5y\cancel{(x+2)}(x+8)} = \dfrac{3(x^2+4)}{5y(x+8)}$

29. $\dfrac{3n^2+15n-18}{3n^2+10n-48} \cdot \dfrac{12n^2-17n-40}{8n^2+2n-10} = \dfrac{3\cancel{(n+6)}\cancel{(n-1)}\cancel{(4n+5)}\cancel{(3n-8)}}{\cancel{(3n-8)}\cancel{(n+6)}2\cancel{(4n+5)}\cancel{(n-1)}} = \dfrac{3}{2}$

33. $\dfrac{x^2-4xy+4y^2}{7xy^2} \div \dfrac{4x^2-3xy-10y^2}{20x^2y+25xy^2} = \dfrac{x^2-4xy+4y^2}{7xy^2} \cdot \dfrac{20x^2y+25xy^2}{4x^2-3xy-10y^2}$

$$= \dfrac{(x-2y)\cancel{(x-2y)}(5\cancel{xy})\cancel{(4x+5y)}}{7\underset{y}{\cancel{xy^2}}\cancel{(4x+5y)}\cancel{(x-2y)}} = \dfrac{5(x-2y)}{7y}$$

37. $\dfrac{3x^4+2x^2-1}{3x^4+14x^2-5} \cdot \dfrac{x^4-2x^2-35}{x^4-17x^2+70} = \dfrac{\cancel{(3x^2-1)}(x^2+1)\cancel{(x^2-7)}\cancel{(x^2+5)}}{\cancel{(3x^2-1)}\cancel{(x^2+5)}\cancel{(x^2-7)}(x^2-10)} = \dfrac{x^2+1}{x^2-10}$

41. $\dfrac{10t^3+25t}{20t+10} \cdot \dfrac{2t^2-t-1}{t^5-t} = \dfrac{\overset{t}{\cancel{5t}}(2t^2+5)(2t+1)\cancel{(t-1)}}{\underset{2}{\cancel{10}}(2t+1)\cancel{(t)}(t+1)\cancel{(t-1)}(t^2+1)} = \dfrac{2t^2+5}{2(t^2+1)(t+1)}$

45. $\dfrac{nr+3n+2r+6}{nr+3n-3r-9} \cdot \dfrac{n^2-9}{n^3-4n} = \dfrac{n(r+3)+2(r+3)}{n(r+3)-3(r+3)} \cdot \dfrac{n^2-9}{n^3-4n} = \dfrac{\cancel{(r+3)}\cancel{(n+2)}(n+3)\cancel{(n-3)}}{\cancel{(r+3)}\cancel{(n-3)}n\cancel{(n+2)}(n-2)} = \dfrac{n+3}{n(n-2)}$

49. $\dfrac{a^2-4ab+4b^2}{6a^2-4ab} \cdot \dfrac{3a^2+5ab-2b^2}{6a^2+ab-b^2} \div \dfrac{a^2-4b^2}{8a+4b}$

Invert the last fraction and multiply.

$$\dfrac{\cancel{(a-2b)}(a-2b)\cancel{(3a-b)}\cancel{(a+2b)}(\overset{2}{\cancel{4}})(2a+b)}{\cancel{2}a(3a-2b)(2a+b)\cancel{(3a-b)}\cancel{(a+2b)}\cancel{(a-2b)}} = \dfrac{2(a-2b)}{a(3a-2b)}$$

Problem Set 4.3

1. $\dfrac{1}{4} + \dfrac{5}{6} = \left(\dfrac{3}{3}\right)\left(\dfrac{1}{4}\right)+\left(\dfrac{2}{2}\right)\left(\dfrac{5}{6}\right) = \dfrac{3}{12} + \dfrac{10}{12} = \dfrac{13}{12}$

5. $\dfrac{6}{5} + \dfrac{1}{-4} = \dfrac{6}{5} - \dfrac{1}{4} = \left(\dfrac{4}{4}\right)\left(\dfrac{6}{5}\right)-\left(\dfrac{5}{5}\right)\left(\dfrac{1}{4}\right) = \dfrac{24}{20} - \dfrac{5}{20} = \dfrac{19}{20}$

9. $\dfrac{1}{5} + \dfrac{5}{6} - \dfrac{7}{15} = \left(\dfrac{6}{6}\right)\left(\dfrac{1}{5}\right)+\left(\dfrac{5}{5}\right)\left(\dfrac{5}{6}\right)-\left(\dfrac{2}{2}\right)\left(\dfrac{7}{15}\right) = \dfrac{6}{30} + \dfrac{25}{30} - \dfrac{14}{30} = \dfrac{17}{30}$

13. $\dfrac{2x}{x-1} + \dfrac{4}{x-1} = \dfrac{2x+4}{x-1}$

17. $\dfrac{3(y-2)}{7y} + \dfrac{4(y-1)}{7y} = \dfrac{3(y-2)+4(y-1)}{7y} = \dfrac{3y-6+4y-4}{7y} = \dfrac{7y-10}{7y}$

21. $\dfrac{2a-1}{4} + \dfrac{3a+2}{6} = \left(\dfrac{3}{3}\right)\left(\dfrac{2a-1}{4}\right)+\left(\dfrac{2}{2}\right)\left(\dfrac{3a+2}{6}\right) = \dfrac{3(2a-1)}{12} + \dfrac{2(3a+2)}{12} = \dfrac{6a-3+6a+4}{12} = \dfrac{12a+1}{12}$

25. $\dfrac{3x-1}{3} - \dfrac{5x+2}{5} = \left(\dfrac{5}{5}\right)\left(\dfrac{3x-1}{3}\right)-\left(\dfrac{3}{3}\right)\left(\dfrac{5x+2}{5}\right) = \dfrac{5(3x-1)}{15} - \dfrac{3(5x+2)}{15} = \dfrac{15x-5-15x-6}{15} = -\dfrac{11}{15}$

29. $\dfrac{3}{8x} + \dfrac{7}{10x} = \left(\dfrac{5}{5}\right)\left(\dfrac{3}{8x}\right)+\left(\dfrac{4}{4}\right)\left(\dfrac{7}{10x}\right) = \dfrac{15}{40x} + \dfrac{28}{40x} = \dfrac{43}{40x}$

33. $\dfrac{4}{3x} + \dfrac{5}{4y} - 1 = \left(\dfrac{4y}{4y}\right)\left(\dfrac{4}{3x}\right)+\left(\dfrac{3x}{3x}\right)\left(\dfrac{5}{4y}\right)-\left(\dfrac{12xy}{12xy}\right)(1)= \dfrac{16y}{12xy} + \dfrac{15x}{12xy} - \dfrac{12xy}{12xy} = \dfrac{16y+15x-12xy}{12xy}$

37. $\dfrac{10}{7n} - \dfrac{12}{4n^2} = \left(\dfrac{4n}{4n}\right)\left(\dfrac{10}{7n}\right)-\left(\dfrac{7}{7}\right)\left(\dfrac{12}{4n^2}\right) = \dfrac{40n}{28n^2} - \dfrac{84}{28n^2} = \dfrac{40n-84}{28n^2} = \dfrac{4(10n-21)}{\underset{7}{28n^2}} = \dfrac{10n-21}{7n^2}$

41. $\dfrac{3}{x} - \dfrac{5}{3x^2} - \dfrac{7}{6x} = \left(\dfrac{6x}{6x}\right)\left(\dfrac{3}{x}\right)-\left(\dfrac{2}{2}\right)\left(\dfrac{5}{3x^2}\right) - \left(\dfrac{x}{x}\right)\left(\dfrac{7}{6x}\right) = \dfrac{18x}{6x^2} - \dfrac{10}{6x^2} - \dfrac{7x}{6x^2}$

$$= \dfrac{18x-10-7x}{6x^2} = \dfrac{11x-10}{6x^2}$$

45. $\dfrac{5b}{24a^2} - \dfrac{11a}{32b} = \left(\dfrac{4b}{4b}\right)\left(\dfrac{5b}{24a^2}\right) - \left(\dfrac{3a^2}{3a^2}\right)\left(\dfrac{11a}{32b}\right) = \dfrac{20b^2}{96a^2b} - \dfrac{33a^3}{96a^2b} = \dfrac{20b^2-33a^3}{96a^2b}$

49. $\dfrac{2x}{x-1} + \dfrac{3}{x} = \left(\dfrac{x}{x}\right)\left(\dfrac{2x}{x-1}\right)+\left(\dfrac{x-1}{x-1}\right)\left(\dfrac{3}{x}\right) = \dfrac{2x^2}{x(x-1)} + \dfrac{3(x-1)}{x(x-1)} = \dfrac{2x^2+3x-3}{x(x-1)}$

53. $\dfrac{-3}{4n-5} - \dfrac{8}{3n+5} = \left(\dfrac{3n+5}{3n+5}\right)\left(\dfrac{-3}{4n+5}\right)-\left(\dfrac{4n+5}{4n+5}\right)\left(\dfrac{8}{3n+5}\right) = \dfrac{-3(3n+5)-8(4n+5)}{(3n+5)(4n+5)}$

$$= \dfrac{-9n-15-32n-40}{(3n+5)(4n+5)} = \dfrac{-41n-55}{(3n+5)(4n+5)}$$

57. $\dfrac{7}{3x-5} - \dfrac{5}{2x+7} = \left(\dfrac{2x+7}{2x+7}\right)\left(\dfrac{7}{3x-5}\right)-\left(\dfrac{3x-5}{3x-5}\right)\left(\dfrac{5}{2x+7}\right) = \dfrac{7(2x+7)-5(3x-5)}{(2x+7)(3x-5)}$

$$= \dfrac{14x+49-15x+25}{(2x+7)(3x-5)} = \dfrac{-x+74}{(2x+7)(3x-5)}$$

61. $\dfrac{3x}{2x+5} + 1 = \dfrac{3x}{2x+5} + \left(\dfrac{2x+5}{2x+5}\right)(1) = \dfrac{3x+(2x+5)}{2x+5} = \dfrac{5x+5}{2x+5}$

65. $-1 - \dfrac{3}{2x+1} = \left(\dfrac{2x+1}{2x+1}\right)(-1) - \dfrac{3}{2x+1} = \dfrac{-(2x+1)-3}{2x+1} = \dfrac{-2x-1-3}{2x+1} = \dfrac{-2x-4}{2x+1}$

Problem Set 4.4

1. $\dfrac{2x}{x^2+4x} + \dfrac{5}{x} = \dfrac{2x}{x(x+4)} + \dfrac{5}{x} = \dfrac{2x}{x(x+9)} + \left(\dfrac{x+4}{x+4}\right)\left(\dfrac{5}{x}\right) = \dfrac{2x+5x+20}{x(x+4)} = \dfrac{7x+20}{x(x+4)}$

5. $\dfrac{x}{x^2-1} + \dfrac{5}{x+1} = \dfrac{x}{(x+1)(x-1)} + \dfrac{5}{x+1} = \dfrac{x}{(x+1)(x-1)} + \left(\dfrac{x-1}{x-1}\right)\left(\dfrac{5}{x+1}\right)$

$$= \dfrac{x+5(x-1)}{(x+1)(x-1)} = \dfrac{x+5x-5}{(x+1)(x-1)} = \dfrac{6x-5}{(x+1)(x-1)}$$

9. $\dfrac{2n}{n^2-25} - \dfrac{3}{4n+20} = \dfrac{2n}{(n+5)(n-5)} - \dfrac{3}{4(n+5)} = \left(\dfrac{4}{4}\right)\left(\dfrac{2n}{(n+5)(n-5)}\right) - \left(\dfrac{n-5}{n-5}\right)\left(\dfrac{3}{4(n+5)}\right)$

$$= \dfrac{8n-3(n-5)}{4(n+5)(n-5)} = \dfrac{8n-3n+15}{4(n+5)(n-5)}$$

$$= \dfrac{5n+15}{4(n+5)(n-5)}$$

13. $\dfrac{3}{x^2+9x+14} + \dfrac{5}{2x^2+15x+7} = \dfrac{3}{(x+7)(x+2)} + \dfrac{5}{(2x+1)(x+7)}$

$$= \left(\dfrac{2x+1}{2x+1}\right)\left(\dfrac{3}{(x+7)(x+2)}\right) + \left(\dfrac{x+2}{x+2}\right)\left(\dfrac{5}{(2x+1)(x+7)}\right)$$

$$= \dfrac{3(2x+1)+5(x+2)}{(2x+1)(x+7)(x+2)} = \dfrac{6x+3+5x+10}{(2x+1)(x+7)(x+2)}$$

$$= \dfrac{11x+13}{(2x+1)(x+7)(x+2)}$$

17. $\dfrac{3a}{20a^2-11a-3} + \dfrac{1}{12a^2+7a-12} = \dfrac{3a}{(5a+1)(4a-3)} + \dfrac{1}{(4a-3)(3a+4)}$

$$= \left(\dfrac{3a+4}{3a+4}\right)\left(\dfrac{3a}{(5a+1)(4a-3)}\right) + \left(\dfrac{5a+1}{5a+1}\right)\left(\dfrac{1}{(4a-5)(3a+4)}\right)$$

$$= \dfrac{3a(3a+4)+1(5a+1)}{(3a+4)(5a+1)(4a-3)} = \dfrac{9a^2+12a+5a+1}{(3a+4)(5a+1)(4a-3)}$$

$$= \dfrac{9a^2+17a+1}{(3a+4)(5a+1)(4a-3)}$$

21. $\dfrac{2}{\underset{(y+8)(y-2)}{\cancel{y^2+6y-16}}} - \dfrac{4}{y+8} - \dfrac{3}{y-2} = \dfrac{2}{(y+8)(y-2)} - \left(\dfrac{y-2}{y-2}\right)\left(\dfrac{4}{y+8}\right) - \left(\dfrac{y+8}{y+8}\right)\left(\dfrac{3}{y-2}\right)$

$$= \dfrac{2-4(y-2)-3(y+8)}{(y+8)(y-2)} = \dfrac{2-4y+8-3y-24}{(y+8)(y-2)} = \dfrac{-7y-14}{(y+8)(y-2)}$$

25. $\dfrac{x+3}{x+10} + \dfrac{4x-3}{\underset{(x+10)(x-2)}{\cancel{x^2+8x-20}}} + \dfrac{x-1}{x-2} = \left(\dfrac{x-2}{x-2}\right)\left(\dfrac{x+3}{x+10}\right) + \dfrac{4x-3}{(x+10)(x-2)} + \left(\dfrac{x+10}{x+10}\right)\left(\dfrac{x-1}{x-2}\right)$

$$= \dfrac{x^2+x-6+4x-3+x^2+9x-10}{(x-2)(x+10)} = \dfrac{2x^2+14x-19}{(x-2)(x+10)}$$

29. $\dfrac{4x-3}{\underset{(2x-1)(x+1)}{\cancel{2x^2+x-1}}} - \dfrac{2x+7}{\underset{(3x-2)(x+1)}{\cancel{3x^2+x-2}}} - \dfrac{3}{3x-2} = \dfrac{(4x-3)(3x-2)-(2x+7)(2x-1)-3(x+1)(2x-1)}{(2x-1)(x+1)(3x-2)}$

$$= \dfrac{12x^2-17x+6-4x^2-12x+7-6x^2-3x+3}{(2x-1)(x+1)(3x-2)}$$

$$= \dfrac{2x^2-32x+16}{(2x-1)(x+1)(3x-2)}$$

33. $\dfrac{\dfrac{15x^2-10}{5x^2-7x+2}}{(5x-2)(x-1)} - \dfrac{3x+4}{x-1} - \dfrac{2}{5x-2} = \dfrac{15x^2-10-(3x+4)(5x-2)-2(x-1)}{(5x-2)(x-1)}$

$$= \dfrac{15x^2-10-15x^2-14x+8-2x+2}{(5x-2)(x-1)} = \dfrac{-16x}{(5x-2)(x-1)}$$

Before doing Problems 37-60, you should review the two basic approaches used in Examples 7 and 8 in Section 4.4 in the text.

37. $\left(\dfrac{\frac{1}{2}-\frac{1}{4}}{\frac{5}{8}+\frac{3}{4}}\right)\left(\dfrac{8}{8}\right) = \dfrac{8(\frac{1}{2})-8(\frac{1}{4})}{8(\frac{5}{8})+8(\frac{3}{4})} = \dfrac{4-2}{5+6} = \dfrac{2}{11}$

41. $\dfrac{\dfrac{5}{6y}}{\dfrac{10}{3xy}} = \left(\dfrac{5}{6y}\right)\left(\dfrac{3xy}{10}\right) = \dfrac{\not{5}\cdot\not{3}\cdot x\cdot\not{y}}{\not{6}\cdot\not{10}\cdot y} = \dfrac{x}{4}$

45. $\left(\dfrac{\frac{6}{a}-\frac{5}{b^2}}{\frac{12}{a^2}+\frac{2}{b}}\right)\left(\dfrac{a^2b^2}{a^2b^2}\right) = \dfrac{\frac{6}{a}(a^2b^2)-\frac{5}{b^2}(a^2b^2)}{\frac{12}{a^2}(a^2b^2)+\frac{2}{b}(a^2b^2)} = \dfrac{6ab^2-5a^2}{12b^2+2a^2b}$

49. $\left(\dfrac{3+\frac{2}{n+4}}{5-\frac{1}{n+4}}\right)\left(\dfrac{n+4}{n+4}\right) = \dfrac{3(n+4)+\frac{2}{n+4}(n+4)}{5(n+4)-\frac{1}{n+4}(n+4)} = \dfrac{3n+12+2}{5n+20-1} = \dfrac{3n+14}{5n+19}$

53. $\left(\dfrac{\frac{-1}{y-2}+\frac{5}{x}}{\frac{3}{x}-\frac{4}{x(y-2)}}\right)\left(\dfrac{x(y-2)}{x(y-2)}\right) = \dfrac{-x+5(y-2)}{3(y-2)-4} = \dfrac{-x+5y-10}{3y-6-4} = \dfrac{-x+5y-10}{3y-10}$

57. $\dfrac{3a}{2-\frac{1}{a}}-1 = \dfrac{3a}{\frac{2a-1}{a}}-1 = (3a)\left(\dfrac{a}{2a-1}\right)-1 = \dfrac{3a^2}{2a-1}-1 = \dfrac{3a^2-1(2a-1)}{2a-1} = \dfrac{3a^2-2a+1}{2a-1}$

Problem Set 4.5

1. $\dfrac{9x^4+18x^3}{3x} = \dfrac{9x^4}{3x}+\dfrac{18x^3}{3x} = 3x^3+6x^2$

5. $\dfrac{15a^3-25a^2-40a}{5a} = \dfrac{15a^3}{5a}-\dfrac{25a^2}{5a}-\dfrac{40a}{5a} = 3a^2-5a-8$

9. $\dfrac{-18x^2y^2+24x^3y^2-48x^2y^3}{6xy} = \dfrac{-18x^2y^2}{6xy}+\dfrac{24x^3y^2}{6xy}-\dfrac{48x^2y^3}{6xy} = -3xy+4x^2y-8xy^2$

13.
$$\begin{array}{r}
x+20 \\
x-8\,\overline{\smash{)}\,x^2+12x-160} \\
\underline{x^2-8x} \\
20x-160 \\
\underline{20x-160}
\end{array}$$

17.
$$\begin{array}{r}
5x-1 \\
3x+5\,\overline{\smash{)}\,15x^2+22x-5} \\
\underline{15x^2+25x} \\
-3x-5 \\
\underline{-3x-5}
\end{array}$$

21.

$$
\begin{array}{r}
x^2 + 5x - 6 \\
2x-1 \overline{\smash{\big)}\, 2x^3+9x^2-17x+6} \\
\underline{2x^3 - x^2} \\
10x^2-17x+6 \\
\underline{10x^2- 5x} \\
-12x+6 \\
\underline{-12x+6}
\end{array}
$$

25.

$$
\begin{array}{r}
x^3 - 4x^2 - 5x + 3 \\
x-6 \overline{\smash{\big)}\, x^4-10x^3+19x^2+33x-18} \\
\underline{x^4- 6x^3} \\
-4x^3+19x^2+33x-18 \\
\underline{-4x^3+24x^2} \\
-5x^2+33x-18 \\
\underline{-5x^2+30x} \\
3x-18 \\
\underline{3x-18}
\end{array}
$$

29.

$$
\begin{array}{r}
x^2 - x + 1 \\
x+1 \overline{\smash{\big)}\, x^3+0x^2+0x+64} \\
\underline{x^3 +x^2} \\
-x^2+0x+64 \\
\underline{-x^2 - x} \\
x+64 \\
\underline{x+ 1} \\
63
\end{array}
$$

33.

$$
\begin{array}{r}
4a - 4b \\
a-b \overline{\smash{\big)}\, 4a^2-8ab+4b^2} \\
\underline{4a^2-4ab} \\
-4ab+4b^2 \\
\underline{-4ab+4b^2}
\end{array}
$$

The following format can also be used.

$$
\begin{array}{r}
x^2 - x + 1 \\
x+1 \overline{\smash{\big)}\, x^3+64} \\
\underline{x^3+x^2} \\
-x^2+64 \\
\underline{-x^2-x} \\
x+64 \\
\underline{x + 1} \\
63
\end{array}
$$

37.

$$
\begin{array}{r}
8y - 9 \\
y^2+y \overline{\smash{\big)}\, 8y^3- y^2- y+5} \\
\underline{8y^3+8y^2} \\
-9y^2- y+5 \\
\underline{-9y^2-9y} \\
8y+5
\end{array}
$$

41.

$$
\begin{array}{r}
x - 3 \\
4x^2-x+5 \overline{\smash{\big)}\, 4x^3-13x^2+8x-15} \\
\underline{4x^3- x^2+5x} \\
-12x^2+3x-15 \\
\underline{-12x^2+3x-15}
\end{array}
$$

45.
$$n^2+1 \overline{\smash{\big)}\,2n^4+3n^3-2n^2+3n-4} \quad 2n^2+3n-4$$

$$2n^4 \qquad +2n^2$$
$$\overline{3n^3-4n^2+3n-4}$$
$$3n^3 \qquad +3n$$
$$\overline{-4n^2 \qquad -4}$$
$$-4n^2 \qquad -4$$

49.
$$x+1 \overline{\smash{\big)}\,x^4+0x^3+0x^2+0x-1} \quad x^3-x^2+x-1$$

$$x^4+ x^3$$
$$\overline{-x^3+0x^2+0x-1}$$
$$-x^3- x^2$$
$$\overline{x^2+0x-1}$$
$$x^2 + x$$
$$\overline{-x-1}$$
$$-x-1$$

Problem Set 4.6

1.
$$\frac{x+1}{4} + \frac{x-2}{6} = \frac{3}{4}$$
$$12\left(\frac{x+1}{4} + \frac{x-2}{6}\right) = 12\left(\frac{3}{4}\right)$$
$$3(x+1)+2(x-2) = 9$$
$$3x+3+2x-4 = 9$$
$$5x-1 = 9$$
$$5x = 10$$
$$x = 2$$

The solution set is $\{2\}$.

5.
$$\frac{5}{n} + \frac{1}{3} = \frac{7}{n}, \quad n \neq 0$$
$$3n\left(\frac{5}{n} + \frac{1}{3}\right) = 3n\left(\frac{7}{n}\right)$$
$$15+n = 21$$
$$n = 6$$

The solution set is $\{6\}$.

9.
$$\frac{3}{4x} + \frac{5}{6} = \frac{4}{3x}, \quad x \neq 0$$
$$12x\left(\frac{3}{4x} + \frac{5}{6}\right) = 12x\left(\frac{4}{3x}\right)$$
$$9+10x = 16$$
$$10x = 7$$
$$x = \frac{7}{10}$$

The solution set is $\left\{\frac{7}{10}\right\}$.

13.
$$\frac{n}{65-n} = 8 + \frac{2}{65-n}, \quad n \neq 65$$
$$(65-n)\left(\frac{n}{65-n}\right) = (65-n)\left(8 + \frac{2}{65-n}\right)$$
$$n = 8(65-n)+2$$
$$n = 520-8n+2$$
$$9n = 522$$
$$n = 58$$

The solution set is $\{58\}$.

17.
$$n - \frac{2}{n} = \frac{23}{5}, \quad n \neq 0$$
$$5n\left(n - \frac{2}{n}\right) = 5n\left(\frac{23}{5}\right)$$
$$5n^2-10 = 23n$$
$$5n^2-23n-10 = 0$$
$$(5n+2)(n-5) = 0$$
$$5n+2 = 0 \quad \text{or} \quad n-5 = 0$$
$$5n = -2 \quad \text{or} \quad n = 5$$
$$n = -\frac{2}{5} \quad \text{or} \quad n = 5$$

The solution set is $\left\{-\frac{2}{5}, 5\right\}$.

21.
$$\frac{-2}{x-5} = \frac{1}{x+9}, \quad x \neq 5 \text{ and } x \neq -9$$
$$1(x-5) = -2(x+9) \quad \text{Apply the cross-multiplication property.}$$
$$x-5 = -2x-18$$
$$3x = -13$$
$$x = -\frac{13}{3}$$

The solution set is $\left\{-\frac{13}{3}\right\}$.

25. $\dfrac{a}{a+5} - 2 = \dfrac{3a}{a+5}$, $a \neq -5$

$$(a+5)(\dfrac{a}{a+5} - 2) = (a+5)(\dfrac{3a}{a+5})$$

$$a - 2(a+5) = 3a$$
$$a - 2a - 10 = 3a$$
$$-a - 10 = 3a$$
$$-10 = 4a$$
$$-\dfrac{10}{4} = a$$
$$-\dfrac{5}{2} = a$$

The solution set is $\{-\dfrac{5}{2}\}$.

29. $\dfrac{3x-7}{10} = \dfrac{2}{x}$, $x \neq 0$

$x(3x-7) = 2(10)$ Apply the cross-multiplication property.

$$3x^2 - 7x = 20$$
$$3x^2 - 7x - 20 = 0$$
$$(3x+5)(x-4) = 0$$
$$3x+5 = 0 \quad \text{or} \quad x-4 = 0$$
$$3x = -5 \text{ or } \quad x = 4$$
$$x = -\dfrac{5}{3} \text{ or } \quad x = 4$$

The solution set is $\{-\dfrac{5}{3}, 4\}$.

33. $\dfrac{3s}{s+2} + 1 = \dfrac{35}{2(3s+1)}$ $s \neq -2$ and $s \neq -\dfrac{1}{3}$

$$[2(s+2)(3s+1)][\dfrac{3s}{s+2} + 1] = [2(s+2)(3s+1)][\dfrac{35}{2(3s+1)}]$$

$$6s(3s+1) + 2(s+2)(3s+1) = 35(s+2)$$
$$18s^2 + 6s + 6s^2 + 14s + 4 = 35s + 70$$
$$24s^2 + 20s + 4 = 35s + 70$$
$$24s^2 - 15s - 66 = 0$$
$$8s^2 - 5s - 22 = 0$$
$$(8s+11)(s-2) = 0$$
$$8s+11 = 0 \quad \text{or } s-2 = 0$$
$$8s = -11 \quad \text{or} \quad s = 2$$
$$x = -\dfrac{11}{8} \quad \text{or} \quad s = 2$$

The solution set is $\{-\dfrac{11}{8}, 2\}$.

37. $\dfrac{n+6}{27} = \dfrac{1}{n}$, $n \neq 0$

$n(n+6) = 27(1)$ Apply the cross-multiplication propery.

$$n^2 + 6n - 27 = 0$$
$$(n+9)(n-3) = 0$$
$$n+9 = 0 \text{ or } n-3 = 0$$
$$n = -9 \text{ or } \quad n = 3$$

The solution set is $\{-9, 3\}$.

41. $\dfrac{-3}{4x+5} = \dfrac{2}{5x-7}$, $x \neq -\dfrac{5}{4}$ and $x \neq \dfrac{7}{5}$

$2(4x+5) = -3(5x-7)$ Apply the cross-multiplication property.
$$8x+10 = -15x+21$$
$$23x = 11$$
$$x = \dfrac{11}{23}$$

The solution set is $\{\dfrac{11}{23}\}$.

45. Let x and 1750-x represent the two sums of money.

$$\frac{x}{1750-x} = \frac{3}{4} \quad , \quad x \neq 1750$$

$$4x = 3(1750-x)$$
$$4x = 5250-3x$$
$$7x = 5250$$
$$x = 750$$

The two sums of money are \$750 and \$1750-\$750 = \$1000.

49. Let n represent the number. Then $\frac{1}{n}$ represents its reciprocal.

$$n + \frac{1}{n} = \frac{53}{14} \quad , \quad n \neq 0$$

$$14n\left(n + \frac{1}{n}\right) = 14n\left(\frac{53}{14}\right)$$

$$14n^2 + 14 = 53n$$

$$14n^2 + 53n + 14 = 0$$
$$(7n-2)(2n-7) = 0$$
$$7n-2 = 0 \text{ or } 2n-7 = 0$$
$$7n = 2 \quad \text{ or } 2n = 7$$
$$n = \frac{2}{7} \quad \text{ or } \quad n = \frac{7}{2}$$

The number is either $\frac{2}{7}$ or $\frac{7}{2}$.

53. Let x represent the amount sold by Laura. Then $120.75 - x$ represents the amount sold by Tammy.

$$\frac{120.75 - x}{x} = \frac{4}{3} \quad , \quad x \neq 0$$

$$4x = 3(120.75 - x)$$
$$4x = 362.25 - 3x$$
$$7x = 362.25$$
$$x = 51.75$$

Tammy's sales amounted to \$51.75 and Laura's sales amounted to \$120.75 - \$51.75 = \$69.

57. Let x and 20-x represent the two lengths.

$$\frac{x}{20-x} = \frac{7}{3} \quad , \quad x \neq 20$$

$$7(20-x) = 3x$$
$$140-7x = 3x$$
$$140 = 10x$$
$$14 = x$$

The board should be cut to produce pieces 14 feet and 20-14 = 6 feet long.

<u>Problem Set 4.7</u>

1.
$$\frac{x}{4(x-1)} + \frac{5}{(x+2)(x-1)} = \frac{1}{4} \quad , \quad x \neq 1 \text{ and } x \neq -2$$

$$[4(x+1)(x-1)][\frac{x}{4(x-1)} + \frac{5}{(x+2)(x-1)}] = [4(x+1)(x-1)][\frac{1}{4}]$$

$$x(x+1)+5(4) = (x+1)(x-1)$$
$$x^2+x+20 = x^2-1$$
$$x = -21$$

The solution set is {-21}.

5.
$$\frac{3}{n-5} + \frac{4}{n+7} = \frac{2n+11}{(n+7)(n-5)} \quad , \quad n \neq 5 \text{ and } n \neq -7$$

$$[(n+7)(n-5)][\frac{3}{n-5} + \frac{4}{n+7}] = [(n+7)(n-5)][\frac{2n+11}{(n+7)(n-5)}]$$

$$3(n+7)+4(n-5) = 2n+11$$
$$3n+21+4n-20 = 2n+11$$
$$7n+1 = 2n+11$$
$$5n = 10$$
$$n = 2$$

The solution set is {2}.

9.
$$1 + \frac{1}{n-1} = \frac{1}{n(n-1)} \quad , \quad n \neq 0 \text{ and } n \neq 1$$

$$n(n-1)[1 + \frac{1}{n-1}] = n(n-1)[\frac{1}{n(n-1)}]$$

$$n(n-1)+n = 1$$
$$n^2-n+n = 1$$
$$n^2-1 = 0$$
$$(n+1)(n-1) = 0$$
$$n+1 = 0 \text{ or } n-1 = 0$$
$$n = -1 \text{ or } \quad n = 1$$

Since the initial restriction was $n \neq 0$ and $n \neq 1$, the solution set is {-1}.

13.
$$\frac{2}{2x-3} - \frac{2}{(2x-3)(5x+1)} = \frac{x}{5x+1} \quad , \quad x \neq \frac{3}{2} \text{ and } x \neq -\frac{1}{5}$$

$$(2x-3)(5x+1)[\frac{2}{2x-3} - \frac{2}{(2x-3)(5x+1)}] = (2x-3)(5x+1)[\frac{x}{5x+1}]$$

$$2(5x+1)-2 = x(2x-3)$$
$$10x+2-2 = 2x^2-3x$$
$$10x = 2x^2-3x$$
$$0 = 2x^2-13x$$
$$0 = x(2x-13)$$
$$x = 0 \text{ or } 2x-13 = 0$$
$$x = 0 \text{ or } \quad 2x = 13$$
$$x = 0 \text{ or } \quad x = \frac{13}{2}$$

The solution set is $\{0, \frac{13}{2}\}$.

17.
$$\frac{a}{a-5} + \frac{2}{a-6} = \frac{2}{(a-5)(a-6)} \quad , \quad a \neq 5 \text{ and } a \neq 6$$

$$(a-5)(a-6)\left[\frac{a}{a-5} + \frac{2}{a-6}\right] = (a-5)(a-6)\left[\frac{2}{(a-5)(a-6)}\right]$$

$$a(a-6)+2(a-5) = 2$$
$$a^2-6a+2a-10 = 2$$
$$a^2-4a-12 = 0$$
$$(a-6)(a+2) = 0$$
$$a-6 = 0 \text{ or } a+2 = 0$$
$$a = 6 \text{ or } a = -2$$

The number 6 cannot be a solution because of the initial restrictions. Thus, the solution set is $\{-2\}$.

21.
$$\frac{7y+2}{(3y+5)(4y-3)} - \frac{1}{3y+5} = \frac{2}{4y-3} \quad , \quad y \neq -\frac{5}{3} \text{ and } y \neq \frac{3}{4}$$

$$(3y+5)(4y-3)\left[\frac{7y+2}{(3y+5)(4y-3)} - \frac{1}{3y+5}\right] = (3y+5)(4y-3)\left[\frac{2}{4y-3}\right]$$

$$7y+2-1(4y-3) = 2(3y+5)$$
$$7y+2-4y+3 = 6y+10$$
$$3y+5 = 6y+10$$
$$-5 = 3y$$
$$-\frac{5}{3} = y$$

Since the initial restriction included $y \neq -\frac{5}{3}$, the solution set is $\varnothing$.

25.
$$\frac{1}{(2x+1)(x-1)} + \frac{3}{x(2x+1)} = \frac{2}{(x+1)(x-1)} \quad , \quad x \neq -\frac{1}{2}, \ x \neq 1, \ x \neq -1, \text{ and } x \neq 0$$

$$x(2x+1)(x+1)(x-1)\left[\frac{1}{(2x+1)(x-1)} + \frac{3}{x(2x+1)}\right] = x(2x+1)(x+1)(x-1)\left[\frac{2}{(x+1)(x-1)}\right]$$

$$x(x+1)+3(x+1)(x-1) = 2x(2x+1)$$
$$x^2+x+3x^2-3 = 4x^2+2x$$
$$x-3 = 2x$$
$$-3 = x$$

The solution set is $\{-3\}$.

29.
$$\frac{4t}{(4t+3)(t-1)} + \frac{2-3t}{(3t+2)(t-1)} = \frac{1}{(4t+3)(3t+2)} \quad , \quad t \neq -\frac{3}{4}, \ t \neq 1, \text{ and } t \neq -\frac{2}{3}$$

Multiply both sides by $(4t+3)(t-1)(3t+2)$.

$$4t(3t+2)+(2-3t)(3+4t) = t-1$$
$$12t^2+8t+6-t-12t^2 = t-1$$
$$7t+6 = t-1$$
$$6t = -7$$
$$t = -\frac{7}{6}$$

The solution set is $\{-\frac{7}{6}\}$.

33.
$$\frac{-2}{x-4} = \frac{5}{y-1}$$

$$-2(y-1) = 5(x-4)$$
$$-2y+2 = 5x-20$$
$$2-5x+20 = 2y$$
$$-5x+22 = 2y$$
$$\frac{-5x+22}{2} = y$$

37.
$$\frac{R}{S} = \frac{T}{S+T}$$

$$R(S+T) = ST$$
$$R = \frac{ST}{S+T}$$

41.
$$\frac{x}{a} + \frac{y}{b} = 1$$

$$\frac{y}{b} = 1 - \frac{x}{a}$$

$$\frac{y}{b} = \frac{a-x}{a}$$

$$y = \frac{b(a-x)}{a} = \frac{ab-bx}{a}$$

45.

	d	r	t
Kent	270	x+4	$\frac{270}{x+4}$
Dave	250	x	$\frac{250}{x}$

Since the times are equal, we can set up and solve the following equation.

$$\frac{270}{x+4} = \frac{250}{x}$$

$$270x = 250(x+4)$$
$$270x = 250x+1000$$
$$20x = 1000$$
$$x = 50$$

Dave drives at 50 miles per hour and Kent drives at 50+4 = 54 miles per hour.

49. Let t represent the time of Katie. Then t-5 represents the time of Connie. Also $\frac{600}{t}$ and $\frac{600}{t-5}$ represent the rates of Katie and Connie, respectively. Since Connie's rate is 20 words per minute faster than Katie's rate, we can set up and solve the following equation.

$$\frac{600}{t-5} = \frac{600}{t} + 20$$

$$t(t-5)\left[\frac{600}{t-5}\right] = t(t-5)\left[\frac{600}{t} + 20\right]$$

$$600t = 600(t-5)+20t(t-5)$$
$$600t = 600t-3000+20t^2-100t$$
$$0 = 20t^2-100t-3000$$
$$0 = t^2-5t-150$$
$$0 = (t-15)(t+10)$$
$$t-15 = 0 \quad \text{or} \quad t+10 = 0$$
$$t = 15 \quad \text{or} \quad t = -10$$

The negative solution must be disregarded; so Katie's time is 15 minutes and Connie's time is 10 minutes. Therefore, Katie's rate is $\frac{600}{15} = 40$ words per minute and Connie's rate is $\frac{600}{10} = 60$ words per minute.

53. Let m represent the number of minutes that it takes Nancy to deliver the
papers. Then 2m represents Amy's time.

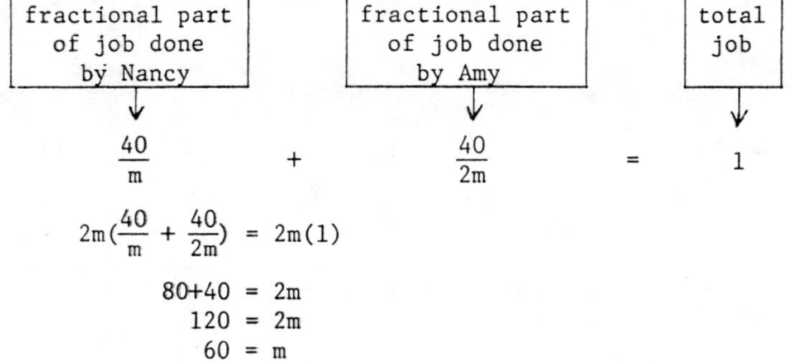

$$2m\left(\frac{40}{m} + \frac{40}{2m}\right) = 2m(1)$$

$$80+40 = 2m$$
$$120 = 2m$$
$$60 = m$$

It would take Nancy 60 minutes and Amy 120 minutes.

57.

	d	r	t
trip out	24	x+4	$\frac{24}{x+4}$
trip back	12	x	$\frac{12}{x}$

Since her return trip took $\frac{1}{2}$ hour less time, the following equation can
be set up and solved.

$$\frac{12}{x} = \frac{24}{x+4} - \frac{1}{2}$$

$$2x(x+4)\left(\frac{12}{x}\right) = 2x(x+4)\left[\frac{24}{x+4} - \frac{1}{2}\right]$$

$$24(x+4) = 2x(24)-x(x+4)$$

$$24x+96 = 48x-x^2-4x$$

$$x^2-20x+96 = 0$$

$$(x-12)(x-8) = 0$$

$$x-12 = 0 \quad \text{or} \quad x-8 = 0$$

$$x = 12 \quad \text{or} \quad x = 8$$

She could ride 16 miles per hour on the way out and 12 miles per hour
back or 12 miles per hour out and 8 miles per hour back.

Chapter 5

<u>Problem Set 5.1</u>

1. $3^{-3} = \dfrac{1}{3^3} = \dfrac{1}{27}$

5. $\dfrac{1}{3^{-4}} = \dfrac{1}{\frac{1}{3^4}} = 3^4 = 81$

9. $\left(-\dfrac{1}{2}\right)^{-3} = \dfrac{1}{\left(-\frac{1}{2}\right)^3} = \dfrac{1}{-\frac{1}{8}} = -8$

13. $\dfrac{1}{\left(\frac{3}{7}\right)^{-2}} = \dfrac{1}{\frac{1}{\left(\frac{3}{7}\right)^2}} = \left(\dfrac{3}{7}\right)^2 = \dfrac{9}{49}$

17. $10^{-5} \cdot 10^2 = 10^{-5+2} = 10^{-3} = \dfrac{1}{10^3} = \dfrac{1}{1000}$

21. $\left(3^{-1}\right)^{-3} = 3^{(-1)(-3)} = 3^3 = 27$

25. $\left(2^3 \cdot 3^{-2}\right)^{-1} = \left(2^3\right)^{-1} \cdot \left(3^{-2}\right)^{-1} = 2^{-3} \cdot 3^2 = \dfrac{1}{2^3} \cdot 9 = \dfrac{1}{8} \cdot 9 = \dfrac{9}{8}$

29. $\left(\dfrac{2^{-1}}{5^{-2}}\right)^{-1} = \dfrac{\left(2^{-1}\right)^{-1}}{\left(5^{-2}\right)^{-1}} = \dfrac{2^1}{5^2} = \dfrac{2}{25}$

33. $\dfrac{3^3}{3^{-1}} = 3^{3-(-1)} = 3^4 = 81$

37. $2^{-2} + 3^{-2} = \dfrac{1}{2^2} + \dfrac{1}{32} = \dfrac{1}{4} + \dfrac{1}{9} = \dfrac{9}{36} + \dfrac{4}{36} = \dfrac{13}{36}$

41. $\left(2^{-3} + 3^{-2}\right)^{-1} = \left(\dfrac{1}{2^3} + \dfrac{1}{3^2}\right)^{-1} = \left(\dfrac{1}{8} + \dfrac{1}{9}\right)^{-1} = \left(\dfrac{17}{72}\right)^{-1} = \dfrac{1}{\left(\frac{17}{72}\right)^1} = \dfrac{72}{17}$

45. $a^3 \cdot a^{-5} \cdot a^{-1} = a^{3+(-5)+(-1)} = a^{-3} = \dfrac{1}{a^3}$

49. $\left(x^2 y^{-6}\right)^{-1} = x^{-2} y^6 = \dfrac{y^6}{x^2}$

53. $\left(2x^3 y^{-4}\right)^{-3} = (2)^{-3}\left(x^3\right)^{-3}\left(y^{-4}\right)^{-3} = 2^{-3} x^{-9} y^{12} = \dfrac{y^{12}}{2^3 x^9} = \dfrac{y^{12}}{8x^9}$

57. $\left(\dfrac{3a^{-2}}{2b^{-1}}\right)^{-2} = \dfrac{(3)^{-2}\left(a^{-2}\right)^{-2}}{(2)^{-2}\left(b^{-1}\right)^{-2}} = \dfrac{3^{-2} a^4}{2^{-2} b^2} = \dfrac{2^2 a^4}{3^2 b^2} = \dfrac{4a^4}{9b^2}$

61. $\dfrac{a^3 b^{-2}}{a^{-2} b^{-4}} = a^{3-(-2)} b^{-2-(-4)} = a^5 b^2$

65. $\left(-7a^2 b^{-5}\right)\left(-a^{-2} b^7\right) = 7a^{2+(-2)} b^{-5+7} = 7a^0 b^2 = 7(1)b^2 = 7b^2$

69. $\dfrac{-72a^2 b^{-4}}{6a^3 b^{-7}} = -12a^{2-3} b^{-4-(-7)} = -12a^{-1} b^3 = -\dfrac{12b^3}{a}$

73. $\left(\dfrac{-36a^{-1}b^{-6}}{4a^{-1}b^{4}}\right)^{-2} = (-9a^{0}b^{-10})^{-2} = (-9b^{-10})^{-2} = (-9)^{-2}(b^{-10})^{-2}$

$$= \dfrac{1}{(-9)^{2}}\,b^{20} = \dfrac{b^{20}}{81}$$

77. $x^{-3} - y^{-1} = \dfrac{1}{x^{3}} - \dfrac{1}{y} = \dfrac{y - x^{3}}{x^{3}y}$

81. $x^{-1}y^{-2} - xy^{-1} = \dfrac{1}{xy^{2}} - \dfrac{x}{y} = \dfrac{1 - x^{2}y}{xy^{2}}$

Problem Set 5.2

1. $\sqrt{64} = 8$ because $8\cdot 8 = 64$

5. $\sqrt[3]{27} = 3$ because $3\cdot 3\cdot 3 = 27$

9. $\sqrt[4]{81} = 3$ because $3\cdot 3\cdot 3\cdot 3 = 81$

13. $-\sqrt{\dfrac{36}{49}} = -\dfrac{6}{7}$

17. $\sqrt[3]{\dfrac{27}{64}} = \dfrac{3}{4}$ because $\dfrac{3}{4}\cdot\dfrac{3}{4}\cdot\dfrac{3}{4} = \dfrac{27}{64}$

21. $\sqrt{27} = \sqrt{9}\sqrt{3} = 3\sqrt{3}$

25. $\sqrt{80} = \sqrt{16}\sqrt{5} = 4\sqrt{5}$

29. $4\sqrt{18} = 4\sqrt{9}\sqrt{2} = 4(3)\sqrt{2} = 12\sqrt{2}$

33. $\dfrac{2}{5}\sqrt{75} = \dfrac{2}{5}\sqrt{25}\sqrt{3} = \dfrac{2}{5}(5)\sqrt{3} = 2\sqrt{3}$

37. $-\dfrac{5}{6}\sqrt{28} = -\dfrac{5}{6}\sqrt{4}\sqrt{7} = -\dfrac{5}{6}(2)\sqrt{7} = -\dfrac{5}{3}\sqrt{7}$

41. $\sqrt{\dfrac{27}{16}} = \dfrac{\sqrt{27}}{\sqrt{16}} = \dfrac{\sqrt{9}\sqrt{3}}{4} = \dfrac{3\sqrt{3}}{4}$

45. $\sqrt{\dfrac{2}{7}} = \sqrt{\dfrac{2}{7}\cdot\dfrac{7}{7}} = \sqrt{\dfrac{14}{49}} = \dfrac{\sqrt{14}}{\sqrt{49}} = \dfrac{\sqrt{14}}{7}$

49. $\dfrac{\sqrt{5}}{\sqrt{12}} = \dfrac{\sqrt{5}}{\sqrt{12}}\cdot\dfrac{\sqrt{3}}{\sqrt{3}} = \dfrac{\sqrt{15}}{\sqrt{36}} = \dfrac{\sqrt{15}}{6}$

53. $\dfrac{\sqrt{18}}{\sqrt{27}} = \sqrt{\dfrac{18}{27}} = \sqrt{\dfrac{2}{3}} = \dfrac{\sqrt{2}}{\sqrt{3}}\cdot\dfrac{\sqrt{3}}{\sqrt{3}} = \dfrac{\sqrt{6}}{3}$

57. $\dfrac{2\sqrt{3}}{\sqrt{7}} = \dfrac{2\sqrt{3}}{\sqrt{7}}\cdot\dfrac{\sqrt{7}}{\sqrt{7}} = \dfrac{2\sqrt{21}}{7}$

61. $\dfrac{3\sqrt{2}}{4\sqrt{3}} = \dfrac{3\sqrt{2}}{4\sqrt{3}}\cdot\dfrac{\sqrt{3}}{\sqrt{3}} = \dfrac{3\sqrt{6}}{4\cdot 3} = \dfrac{\sqrt{6}}{4}$

65. $\sqrt[3]{16} = \sqrt[3]{8}\,\sqrt[3]{2} = 2\sqrt[3]{2}$

69. $\dfrac{2}{\sqrt[3]{9}} = \dfrac{2}{\sqrt[3]{9}}\cdot\dfrac{\sqrt[3]{3}}{\sqrt[3]{3}} = \dfrac{2\sqrt[3]{3}}{3}$

73. $\dfrac{\sqrt[3]{6}}{\sqrt[3]{4}} = \dfrac{\sqrt[3]{6}}{\sqrt[3]{4}}\cdot\dfrac{\sqrt[3]{2}}{\sqrt[3]{2}} = \dfrac{\sqrt[3]{12}}{2}$

Problem Set 5.3

1. $5\sqrt{18} - 2\sqrt{2} = 5\sqrt{9}\sqrt{2} - 2\sqrt{2} = 5(3)\sqrt{2} - 2\sqrt{2} = 15\sqrt{2} - 2\sqrt{2} = 13\sqrt{2}$

5. $-2\sqrt{50} - 5\sqrt{32} = -2\sqrt{25}\sqrt{2} - 5\sqrt{16}\sqrt{2} = -2(5)\sqrt{2} - 5(4)\sqrt{2} = -10\sqrt{2} - 20\sqrt{2} = -30\sqrt{2}$

9. $-9\sqrt{24} + 3\sqrt{54} - 12\sqrt{6} = -9\sqrt{4}\sqrt{6} + 3\sqrt{9}\sqrt{6} - 12\sqrt{6} = -9(2)\sqrt{6} + 3(3)\sqrt{6} - 12\sqrt{6}$

$$= -18\sqrt{6} + 9\sqrt{6} - 12\sqrt{6} = -21\sqrt{6}$$

13. $\dfrac{3}{5}\sqrt{40} + \dfrac{5}{6}\sqrt{90} = \dfrac{3}{5}\sqrt{4}\sqrt{10} + \dfrac{5}{6}\sqrt{9}\sqrt{10} = \dfrac{3}{5}(2)\sqrt{10} + \dfrac{5}{6}(3)\sqrt{10} = \dfrac{6}{5}\sqrt{10} + \dfrac{5}{2}\sqrt{10}$

$$= \left(\dfrac{6}{5} + \dfrac{5}{2}\right)\sqrt{10} = \dfrac{37}{10}\sqrt{10}$$

17. $5\sqrt[3]{3} + 2\sqrt[3]{24} - 6\sqrt[3]{81} = 5\sqrt[3]{3} + 2\sqrt[3]{8}\sqrt[3]{3} - 6\sqrt[3]{27}\sqrt[3]{3} = 5\sqrt[3]{3} + 2(2)\sqrt[3]{3} - 6(3)\sqrt[3]{3}$

$$= 5\sqrt[3]{3} + 4\sqrt[3]{3} - 18\sqrt[3]{3} = -9\sqrt[3]{3}$$

21. $\sqrt{32x} = \sqrt{16}\sqrt{2x} = 4\sqrt{2x}$ 25. $\sqrt{20x^2y} = \sqrt{4x^2}\sqrt{5y} = 2x\sqrt{5y}$

29. $\sqrt{54a^4b^3} = \sqrt{9a^4b^2}\sqrt{6b} = 3a^2b\sqrt{6b}$

33. $2\sqrt{40a^3} = 2\sqrt{4a^2}\sqrt{10a} = 2(2a)\sqrt{10a} = 4a\sqrt{10a}$

37. $\sqrt{\dfrac{2x}{5y}} = \sqrt{\dfrac{2x}{5y} \cdot \dfrac{5y}{5y}} = \sqrt{\dfrac{10xy}{25y^2}} = \dfrac{\sqrt{10xy}}{\sqrt{25y^2}} = \dfrac{\sqrt{10xy}}{5y}$

41. $\dfrac{5}{\sqrt{18y}} = \dfrac{5}{\sqrt{18y}} \cdot \dfrac{\sqrt{2y}}{\sqrt{2y}} = \dfrac{5\sqrt{2y}}{\sqrt{36y^2}} = \dfrac{5\sqrt{2y}}{6y}$

45. $\dfrac{\sqrt{18y^3}}{\sqrt{16x}} = \dfrac{\sqrt{9y^2}\sqrt{2y}}{\sqrt{16}\sqrt{x}} = \dfrac{3y\sqrt{2y}}{4\sqrt{x}} = \dfrac{3y\sqrt{2y}}{4\sqrt{x}} \cdot \dfrac{\sqrt{x}}{\sqrt{x}} = \dfrac{3y\sqrt{2xy}}{4x}$

49. $\sqrt[3]{24y} = \sqrt[3]{8}\sqrt[3]{3y} = 2\sqrt[3]{3y}$ 53. $\sqrt[3]{56x^6y^8} = \sqrt[3]{8x^6y^6}\sqrt[3]{7y^2} = 2x^2y^2\sqrt[3]{7y^2}$

57. $\dfrac{\sqrt[3]{3y}}{\sqrt[3]{16x^4}} = \dfrac{\sqrt[3]{3y}}{\sqrt[3]{8x^3}\sqrt[3]{2x}} = \dfrac{\sqrt[3]{3y}}{2x\sqrt[3]{2x}} = \dfrac{\sqrt[3]{3y}}{2x\sqrt[3]{2x}} \cdot \dfrac{\sqrt[3]{4x^2}}{\sqrt[3]{4x^2}} = \dfrac{\sqrt[3]{12x^2y}}{2x(2x)} = \dfrac{\sqrt[3]{12x^2y}}{4x^2}$

61. $\sqrt{8x+12y} = \sqrt{4(2x+3y)} = \sqrt{4}\sqrt{2x+3y} = 2\sqrt{2x+3y}$

65. $-3\sqrt{4x} + 5\sqrt{9x} + 6\sqrt{16x} = -3\sqrt{4}\sqrt{x} + 5\sqrt{9}\sqrt{x} + 6\sqrt{16}\sqrt{x} = -3(2)\sqrt{x} + 5(3)\sqrt{x} + 6(4)\sqrt{x}$
$$= -6\sqrt{x} + 15\sqrt{x} + 24\sqrt{x} = 33\sqrt{x}$$

69. $5\sqrt{27n} - \sqrt{12n} - 6\sqrt{3n} = 5\sqrt{9}\sqrt{3n} - \sqrt{4}\sqrt{3n} - 6\sqrt{3n} = 5(3)\sqrt{3n} - 2\sqrt{3n} - 6\sqrt{3n}$
$$= 15\sqrt{3n} - 2\sqrt{3n} - 6\sqrt{3n} = 7\sqrt{3n}$$

73. $-3\sqrt{2x^3} + 4\sqrt{8x^3} - 3\sqrt{32x^3} = -3\sqrt{x^2}\sqrt{2x} + 4\sqrt{4x^2}\sqrt{2x} - 3\sqrt{16x^2}\sqrt{2x}$
$$= -3x\sqrt{2x} + 4(2x)\sqrt{2x} - 3(4x)\sqrt{2x}$$
$$= -3x\sqrt{2x} + 8x\sqrt{2x} - 12x\sqrt{2x} = -7x\sqrt{2x}$$

<u>Problem Set 5.4</u>

1. $\sqrt{6}\sqrt{12} = \sqrt{72} = \sqrt{36}\sqrt{2} = 6\sqrt{2}$ 5. $(4\sqrt{2})(-6\sqrt{5}) = -24\sqrt{10}$

9. $(5\sqrt{6})(4\sqrt{6}) = 20(6) = 120$

13. $(4\sqrt[3]{6})(7\sqrt[3]{4}) = 28\sqrt[3]{24} = 28\sqrt[3]{8}\sqrt[3]{3} = 28(2)\sqrt[3]{3} = 56\sqrt[3]{3}$

17. $3\sqrt{5}(2\sqrt{2} - \sqrt{7}) = (3\sqrt{5})(2\sqrt{2}) - (3\sqrt{5})(\sqrt{7}) = 6\sqrt{10} - 3\sqrt{35}$

21. $-4\sqrt{5}(2\sqrt{5} + 4\sqrt{12}) = (-4\sqrt{5})(2\sqrt{5}) + (-4\sqrt{5})(4\sqrt{12}) = -8(5) - 16\sqrt{60}$
$$= -40 - 16\sqrt{4}\sqrt{15} = -40 - 32\sqrt{15}$$

25. $\sqrt{xy}(5\sqrt{xy} - 6\sqrt{x}) = (\sqrt{xy})(5\sqrt{xy}) - (\sqrt{xy})(6\sqrt{x}) = 5xy - 6x\sqrt{y}$

29. $5\sqrt{3}(2\sqrt{8} - 3\sqrt{18}) = (5\sqrt{3})(2\sqrt{8}) - (5\sqrt{3})(3\sqrt{18}) = 10\sqrt{24} - 15\sqrt{54}$
$$= 10\sqrt{4}\sqrt{6} - 15\sqrt{9}\sqrt{6}$$
$$= 20\sqrt{6} - 45\sqrt{6} = -25\sqrt{6}$$

33. $(\sqrt{5} - 6)(\sqrt{5} - 3) = \sqrt{5}(\sqrt{5} - 3) - 6(\sqrt{5} - 3) = 5 - 3\sqrt{5} - 6\sqrt{5} + 18 = 23 - 9\sqrt{5}$

37. $(2\sqrt{6} + 3\sqrt{5})(\sqrt{8} - 3\sqrt{12}) = 2\sqrt{6}(\sqrt{8} - 3\sqrt{12}) + 3\sqrt{5}(\sqrt{8} - 3\sqrt{12})$

$$= 2\sqrt{48} - 6\sqrt{72} + 3\sqrt{40} - 9\sqrt{60}$$

$$= 2\sqrt{16}\sqrt{3} - 6\sqrt{36}\sqrt{2} + 3\sqrt{4}\sqrt{10} - 9\sqrt{4}\sqrt{15}$$

$$= 8\sqrt{3} - 36\sqrt{2} + 6\sqrt{10} - 18\sqrt{15}$$

41. $(3\sqrt{2} - 5\sqrt{3})(6\sqrt{2} - 7\sqrt{3}) = 3\sqrt{2}(6\sqrt{2} - 7\sqrt{3}) - 5\sqrt{3}(6\sqrt{2} - 7\sqrt{3})$

$$= 18(2) - 21\sqrt{6} - 30\sqrt{6} + 35(3) = 36 - 51\sqrt{6} + 105 = 141 - 51\sqrt{6}$$

45. Apply the pattern $(a+b)(a-b) = a^2 - b^2$.

$$(\sqrt{2} + \sqrt{10})(\sqrt{2} - \sqrt{10}) = (\sqrt{2})^2 - (\sqrt{10})^2 = 2 - 10 = -8$$

49. $2\sqrt[3]{3}(5\sqrt[3]{4} + \sqrt[3]{6}) = 10\sqrt[3]{12} + 2\sqrt[3]{18}$

53. $\dfrac{2}{\sqrt{7} + 1} = \left(\dfrac{2}{\sqrt{7} + 1}\right)\left(\dfrac{\sqrt{7} - 1}{\sqrt{7} - 1}\right) = \dfrac{2(\sqrt{7} - 1)}{7 - 1} = \dfrac{2(\sqrt{7} - 1)}{6} = \dfrac{\sqrt{7} - 1}{3}$

57. $\dfrac{1}{\sqrt{2} + \sqrt{7}} = \left(\dfrac{1}{\sqrt{2} + \sqrt{7}}\right)\left(\dfrac{\sqrt{2} - \sqrt{7}}{\sqrt{2} - \sqrt{7}}\right) = \dfrac{\sqrt{2} - \sqrt{7}}{2 - 7} = \dfrac{\sqrt{2} - \sqrt{7}}{-5} = \dfrac{\sqrt{7} - \sqrt{2}}{5}$

61. $\dfrac{\sqrt{3}}{2\sqrt{5} + 4} = \left(\dfrac{3}{2\sqrt{5} + 4}\right)\left(\dfrac{2\sqrt{5} - 4}{2\sqrt{5} - 4}\right) = \dfrac{2\sqrt{15} - 4\sqrt{3}}{20 - 16} = \dfrac{2(\sqrt{15} - 2\sqrt{3})}{4} = \dfrac{\sqrt{15} - 2\sqrt{3}}{2}$

65. $\dfrac{\sqrt{6}}{3\sqrt{2} + 2\sqrt{3}} = \left(\dfrac{\sqrt{6}}{3\sqrt{2} + 2\sqrt{3}}\right)\left(\dfrac{3\sqrt{2} - 2\sqrt{3}}{3\sqrt{2} - 2\sqrt{3}}\right) = \dfrac{3\sqrt{12} - 2\sqrt{18}}{18 - 12} = \dfrac{6\sqrt{3} - 6\sqrt{2}}{6}$

$$= \dfrac{6(\sqrt{3} - \sqrt{2})}{6} = \sqrt{3} - \sqrt{2}$$

69. $\dfrac{\sqrt{x}}{\sqrt{x} - 5} = \left(\dfrac{\sqrt{x}}{\sqrt{x} - 5}\right)\left(\dfrac{\sqrt{x} + 5}{\sqrt{x} + 5}\right) = \dfrac{x + 5\sqrt{x}}{x - 25}$

73. $\dfrac{\sqrt{x}}{\sqrt{x} + 2\sqrt{y}} = \left(\dfrac{\sqrt{x}}{\sqrt{x} + 2\sqrt{y}}\right)\left(\dfrac{\sqrt{x} - 2\sqrt{y}}{\sqrt{x} - 2\sqrt{y}}\right) = \dfrac{x - 2\sqrt{xy}}{x - 4y}$

Problem Set 5.5

Don't forget that you <u>must</u> <u>check</u> your answers in this section to eliminate any extraneous roots.

1.
$$\sqrt{5x} = 10$$

$(\sqrt{5x})^2 = (10)^2$ Square both sides.

$$5x = 100$$
$$x = 20$$

Check

$$\sqrt{5x} = 10$$
$$\sqrt{5(20)} \overset{?}{=} 10$$
$$\sqrt{100} \overset{?}{=} 10$$
$$10 = 10$$

The solution set is $\{20\}$.

5.
$$2\sqrt{n} = 5$$
$$(2\sqrt{n})^2 = (5)^2 \quad \text{Square both sides.}$$
$$4n = 25$$
$$n = \frac{25}{4}$$

Check
$$2\sqrt{n} = 5$$
$$2\sqrt{\frac{25}{4}} \stackrel{?}{=} 5$$
$$2\left(\frac{5}{2}\right) \stackrel{?}{=} 5$$
$$5 = 5$$

The solution set is $\{\frac{25}{4}\}$.

9.
$$\sqrt{3y+1} = 4$$
$$(\sqrt{3y+1})^2 = (4)^2 \quad \text{Square both sides.}$$
$$3y+1 = 16$$
$$3y = 15$$
$$y = 5$$

Check
$$\sqrt{3y+1} = 4$$
$$\sqrt{3(5)+1} \stackrel{?}{=} 4$$
$$\sqrt{16} \stackrel{?}{=} 4$$
$$4 = 4$$

The solution set is $\{5\}$.

13. The expression $\sqrt{2x-5}$ will always be nonnegative; therefore, it cannot equal -1. The solution set is $\emptyset$.

17.
$$\sqrt{3x+1} = \sqrt{7x-5}$$
$$(\sqrt{3x+1})^2 = (\sqrt{7x-5})^2 \quad \text{Square both sides.}$$
$$3x+1 = 7x-5$$
$$6 = 4x$$
$$\frac{6}{4} = x$$
$$\frac{3}{2} = x$$

Check
$$\sqrt{3x+1} = \sqrt{7x-5}$$
$$\sqrt{3\left(\frac{3}{2}\right)+1} \stackrel{?}{=} \sqrt{7\left(\frac{3}{2}\right)-5}$$
$$\sqrt{\frac{9}{2}+1} \stackrel{?}{=} \sqrt{\frac{21}{2}-5}$$
$$\sqrt{\frac{11}{2}} = \sqrt{\frac{11}{2}}$$

The solution set is $\{\frac{3}{2}\}$.

21.
$$5\sqrt{t-1} = 6$$
$$(5\sqrt{t-1})^2 = (6)^2 \quad \text{Square both sides.}$$
$$25(t-1) = 36$$
$$25t-25 = 36$$
$$25t = 61$$
$$t = \frac{61}{25}$$

Check
$$5\sqrt{t-1} = 6$$
$$5\sqrt{\frac{61}{25}-1} \stackrel{?}{=} 6$$
$$5\sqrt{\frac{36}{25}} \stackrel{?}{=} 6$$
$$5\left(\frac{6}{5}\right) \stackrel{?}{=} 6$$
$$6 = 6$$

The solution set is $\{\frac{61}{25}\}$.

25. $\quad\sqrt{x^2+13x+37} = 1$

$\quad(\sqrt{x^2+13x+37})^2 = (1)^2$ Square both sides.

$\quad\quad x^2+13x+37 = 1$

$\quad\quad x^2+13x+36 = 0$

$\quad\quad (x+4)(x+9) = 0$

$\quad\quad x+4 = 0 \ \text{ or } \ x+9 = 0$

$\quad\quad\quad x = -4 \text{ or } \quad x = -9$

Check

$$\sqrt{x^2+13x+37} = 1$$

$\sqrt{(-4)^2+13(-4)+37} \overset{?}{=} 1 \qquad\qquad \sqrt{(-9)^2+13(-9)+37} \overset{?}{=} 1$

$\quad\quad \sqrt{16-52+37} \overset{?}{=} 1 \qquad\qquad\quad \sqrt{81-117+37} \overset{?}{=} 1$

$\quad\quad\quad\quad\quad \sqrt{1} \overset{?}{=} 1 \qquad\qquad\qquad\quad \sqrt{118-117} \overset{?}{=} 1$

$\quad\quad\quad\quad\quad 1 = 1 \qquad\qquad\qquad\qquad\quad \sqrt{1} = 1$

$\quad\quad\quad\quad\qquad\qquad\qquad\qquad\qquad\qquad\quad 1 = 1$

The solution set is $\{-9,-4\}$.

29. $\quad\sqrt{x^2+3x+7} = x+2$

$\quad(\sqrt{x^2+3x+7})^2 = (x+2)^2$ Square both sides.

$\quad\quad x^2+3x+7 = x^2+4x+4$

$\quad\quad\quad\quad\quad 3 = x$

Check

$$\sqrt{x^2+3x+7} = x+2$$

$\sqrt{3^2+3(3)+7} \overset{?}{=} 3+2$

$\quad\quad\quad \sqrt{25} \overset{?}{=} 5$

$\quad\quad\quad\quad 5 = 5$

The solution set is $\{3\}$.

33. $\quad\sqrt{n+4} = n+4$

$\quad(\sqrt{n+4})^2 = (n+4)^2$ Square both sides.

$\quad\quad n+4 = n^2+8n+16$

$\quad\quad\quad 0 = n^2+7n+12$

$\quad\quad\quad 0 = (n+3)(n+4)$

$\quad\quad n+3 = 0 \ \text{ or } \ n+4 = 0$

$\quad\quad\quad n = -3 \text{ or } \quad n = -4$

Check $\quad\quad \sqrt{n+4} = n+4$

$\sqrt{-3+4} \overset{?}{=} -3+4 \qquad \sqrt{-4+4} \overset{?}{=} -4+4$

$\quad\quad \sqrt{1} \overset{?}{=} 1 \qquad\qquad\quad \sqrt{0} \overset{?}{=} 0$

$\quad\quad\quad 1 = 1 \qquad\qquad\qquad 0 = 0$

The solution set is $\{-4,-3\}$.

37. $\quad 4\sqrt{x}+5 = x$

$\quad\quad 4\sqrt{x} = x-5$

$\quad (4\sqrt{x})^2 = (x-5)^2$ Square both sides.

$\quad\quad 16x = x^2-10x+25$

$\quad\quad\quad 0 = x^2-26x+25$

$\quad\quad\quad 0 = (x-25)(x-1)$

$\quad x-25 = 0 \ \text{ or } \ x-1 = 0$

$\quad\quad x = 25 \text{ or } \quad x = 1$

Check $\quad\quad 4\sqrt{x}+5 = x$

$4\sqrt{25}+5 \overset{?}{=} 25 \qquad 4\sqrt{1}+5 \overset{?}{=} 1$

$\quad 4(5)+5 \overset{?}{=} 25 \qquad\quad 4+5 \overset{?}{=} 1$

$\quad\quad\quad 25 = 25 \qquad\qquad\quad 9 \neq 1$

The solution set is $\{25\}$.

41. $\sqrt[3]{2x+3} = -3$

$(\sqrt[3]{2x+3})^3 = (-3)^3$ Cube both sides.

$2x+3 = -27$

$2x = -30$

$x = -15$

Check

$\sqrt[3]{2x+3} = -3$

$\sqrt[3]{2(-15)+3} \overset{?}{=} -3$

$\sqrt[3]{-27} \overset{?}{=} -3$

$-3 = -3$

The solution set is $\{-15\}$.

45. $\sqrt{x+19} - \sqrt{x+28} = -1$

$\sqrt{x+19} = \sqrt{x+28} - 1$

$(\sqrt{x+19})^2 = (\sqrt{x+28} - 1)^2$ Square both sides.

$x+19 = x+28 - 2\sqrt{x+28} + 1$

$x+19 = x+29 - 2\sqrt{x+28}$

$-10 = -2\sqrt{x+28}$

$5 = \sqrt{x+28}$

$(5)^2 = (\sqrt{x+28})^2$ Square both sides again.

$25 = x+28$

$-3 = x$

Check

$\sqrt{x+19} - \sqrt{x+28} = -1$

$\sqrt{-3+19} - \sqrt{-3+28} \overset{?}{=} -1$

$\sqrt{16} - \sqrt{25} \overset{?}{=} -1$

$4 - 5 \overset{?}{=} -1$

$-1 = -1$

The solution set is $\{-3\}$.

49. $\sqrt{n-4} + \sqrt{n+4} = 2\sqrt{n-1}$

$(\sqrt{n-4} + \sqrt{n+4})^2 = (2\sqrt{n-1})^2$ Square both sides.

$n-4 + 2\sqrt{n^2-16} + n+4 = 4(n-1)$

$2\sqrt{n^2-16} + 2n = 4(n-1)$

$2(\sqrt{n^2-16} + n) = 4(n-1)$

$\sqrt{n^2-16} + n = 2n-2$

$\sqrt{n^2-16} = n-2$

$(\sqrt{n^2-16})^2 = (n-2)^2$ Square both sides again.

$n^2-16 = n^2-4n+4$

$4n = 20$

$n = 5$

Check

$\sqrt{n-4} + \sqrt{n+4} = 2\sqrt{n-1}$

$\sqrt{5-4} + \sqrt{5+4} \overset{?}{=} 2\sqrt{5-1}$

$\sqrt{1} + \sqrt{9} \overset{?}{=} 2\sqrt{4}$

$1+3 = 4$

$4 = 4$

The solution set is $\{5\}$.

<u>Problem Set 5.6</u>

1. $81^{\frac{1}{2}} = \sqrt{81} = 9$

5. $(-8)^{\frac{1}{3}} = \sqrt[3]{-8} = -2$

9. $36^{-\frac{1}{2}} = \dfrac{1}{36^{\frac{1}{2}}} = \dfrac{1}{\sqrt{36}} = \dfrac{1}{6}$

13. $4^{\frac{3}{2}} = (\sqrt{4})^3 = 2^3 = 8$

17. $(-1)^{\frac{7}{3}} = (\sqrt[3]{-1})^7 = (-1)^7 = -1$

21. $\left(\dfrac{27}{8}\right)^{\frac{4}{3}} = \left(\sqrt[3]{\dfrac{27}{8}}\right)^4 = \left(\dfrac{3}{2}\right)^4 = \dfrac{81}{16}$

25. $(64)^{-\frac{7}{6}} = \dfrac{1}{(64)^{\frac{7}{6}}} = \dfrac{1}{(\sqrt[6]{64})^7} = \dfrac{1}{2^7} = \dfrac{1}{128}$

29. $125^{\frac{4}{3}} = (\sqrt[3]{125})^4 = 5^4 = 625$

33. $3x^{\frac{1}{2}} = 3\sqrt{x}$

37. $(2x-3y)^{\frac{1}{2}} = \sqrt{2x-3y}$

41. $x^{\frac{2}{3}}y^{\frac{1}{3}} = \sqrt[3]{x^2 y}$

45. $\sqrt{5y} = (5y)^{\frac{1}{2}} = 5^{\frac{1}{2}}y^{\frac{1}{2}}$

49. $\sqrt[3]{xy^2} = x^{\frac{1}{3}}y^{\frac{2}{3}}$

53. $\sqrt[5]{(2x-y)^3} = (2x-y)^{\frac{3}{5}}$

57. $-\sqrt[3]{x+y} = -(x+y)^{\frac{1}{3}}$

61. $(y^{\frac{2}{3}})(y^{-\frac{1}{4}}) = y^{\frac{2}{3}+(-\frac{1}{4})} = y^{\frac{8}{12}-\frac{3}{12}} = y^{\frac{5}{12}}$

65. $\left(4x^{\frac{1}{2}}y\right)^2 = (4)^2\left(x^{\frac{1}{2}}\right)^2(y)^2 = 16xy^2$

69. $\dfrac{24x^{\frac{3}{5}}}{6x^{\frac{1}{3}}} = 4x^{\frac{3}{5}-\frac{1}{3}} = 4x^{\frac{9}{15}-\frac{5}{15}} = 4x^{\frac{4}{15}}$

73. $\left(\dfrac{6x^{\frac{2}{5}}}{7y^{\frac{2}{3}}}\right)^2 = \dfrac{(6)^2\left(x^{\frac{2}{5}}\right)^2}{(7)^2\left(y^{\frac{2}{3}}\right)^2} = \dfrac{36x^{\frac{4}{5}}}{49y^{\frac{4}{3}}}$

77. $\left(\dfrac{18x^{\frac{1}{3}}}{9x^{\frac{1}{4}}}\right)^2 = \left(2x^{\frac{1}{3}-\frac{1}{4}}\right)^2 = \left(2x^{\frac{1}{12}}\right)^2 = (2)^2\left(x^{\frac{1}{12}}\right)^2 = 4x^{\frac{2}{12}} = 4x^{\frac{1}{6}}$

81. $\sqrt[3]{3}\,\sqrt{3} = 3^{\frac{1}{3}} \cdot 3^{\frac{1}{2}} = 3^{\frac{1}{3}+\frac{1}{2}} = 3^{\frac{5}{6}} = \sqrt[6]{3^5} = \sqrt[6]{243}$

85. $\dfrac{\sqrt[3]{3}}{\sqrt[4]{3}} = \dfrac{3^{\frac{1}{3}}}{3^{\frac{1}{4}}} = 3^{\frac{1}{3}-\frac{1}{4}} = 3^{\frac{1}{12}} = \sqrt[12]{3}$

89. $\dfrac{\sqrt[4]{27}}{\sqrt{3}} = \dfrac{\sqrt[4]{3^3}}{\sqrt{3}} = \dfrac{3^{\frac{3}{4}}}{3^{\frac{1}{2}}} = 3^{\frac{3}{4}-\frac{1}{2}} = 3^{\frac{1}{4}} = \sqrt[4]{3}$

<u>Problem Set 5.7</u>

For Problems 1-18, refer to the text for the specific procedure for changing from ordinary notation to scientific notation.

For Problems 19-32, refer to the text for the specific procedure for changing from scientific notation to ordinary notation.

33. $(.0037)(.00002) = (3.7)(10^{-3})(2)(10^{-5}) = (7.4)(10^{-8}) = .000000074$

37. $\dfrac{360,000,000}{.0012} = \dfrac{(3.6)(10^{8})}{(1.2)(10^{-3})} = (3)(10^{11}) = 300,000,000,000$

41. $\dfrac{(60,000)(.006)}{(.0009)(400)} = \dfrac{(6)(10^{4})(6)(10^{-3})}{(9)(10^{-4})(4)(10^{2})} = \dfrac{(36)(10)}{(36)(10^{-2})} = (1)(10^{3}) = 1000$

45. $\sqrt{9,000,000} = \sqrt{(9)(10^{6})} = \sqrt{9}\sqrt{10^{6}} = (3)(10^{3}) = 3000$

49. $(90,000)^{\frac{3}{2}} = [(9)(10^{4})]^{\frac{3}{2}} = (9)^{\frac{3}{2}}(10^{4})^{\frac{3}{2}} = 27(10^{6}) = 27,000,000$

<u>Problem Set 6.1</u>

1. $x^2-9x = 0$
$x(x-9) = 0$
$x = 0$ or $x-9 = 0$
$x = 0$ or $x = 9$

The solution set is $\{0,9\}$.

5. $3y^2+12y = 0$
$3y(y+4) = 0$
$3y = 0$ or $y+4 = 0$
$y = 0$ or $y = -4$

The solution set is $\{-4,0\}$.

9. $x^2+x-30 = 0$
$(x+6)(x-5) = 0$
$x+6 = 0$ or $x-5 = 0$
$x = -6$ or $x = 5$

The solution set is $\{-6,5\}$.

13. $2x^2+19x+24 = 0$
$(2x+3)(x+8) = 0$
$2x+3 = 0$ or $x+8 = 0$
$2x = -3$ or $x = -8$
$x = -\dfrac{3}{2}$ or $x = -8$

The solution set is $\{-8, -\dfrac{3}{2}\}$.

17. $25x^2-30x+9 = 0$
$(5x-3)(5x-3) = 0$
$5x-3 = 0$ or $5x-3 = 0$
$5x = 3$ or $5x = 3$
$x = \dfrac{3}{5}$ or $x = \dfrac{3}{5}$

The solution set is $\{\dfrac{3}{5}\}$.

21. $3\sqrt{x} = x+2$
$(3\sqrt{x})^2 = (x+2)^2$ Square both sides.
$9x = x^2+4x+4$
$0 = x^2-5x+4$
$0 = (x-4)(x-1)$
$x-4 = 0$ or $x-1 = 0$
$x = 4$ or $x = 1$

<u>Check</u> $\quad 3\sqrt{x} = x+2$

$3\sqrt{4} \stackrel{?}{=} 4+2 \qquad 3\sqrt{1} \stackrel{?}{=} 1+2$
$3(2) \stackrel{?}{=} 4+2 \qquad 3(1) \stackrel{?}{=} 1+2$
$6 = 6 \qquad\qquad 3 = 3$

The solution set is $\{1,4\}$.

25. $\sqrt{3x}+6 = x$
$\sqrt{3x} = x-6$
$(\sqrt{3x})^2 = (x-6)^2$ Square both sides.
$3x = x^2-12x+36$
$0 = x^2-15x+36$
$0 = (x-12)(x-3)$
$x-12 = 0$ or $x-3 = 0$
$x = 12$ or $x = 3$

The solution set is $\{12\}$.

<u>Check</u> $\quad \sqrt{3x}+6 = x$

$\sqrt{3(12)}+6 \stackrel{?}{=} 12 \qquad \sqrt{3(3)}+6 \stackrel{?}{=} 3$
$\sqrt{36}+6 \stackrel{?}{=} 12 \qquad \sqrt{9}+6 \stackrel{?}{=} 3$
$6+6 = 12 \qquad\qquad 3+6 \neq 3$

29.
$$x^2 = 16k^2 x$$
$$x^2 - 16k^2 x = 0$$
$$x(x - 16k^2) = 0$$
$$x = 0 \text{ or } x - 16k^2 = 0$$
$$x = 0 \text{ or } \quad x = 16k^2$$

The solution set is $\{0, 16k^2\}$.

37.
$$6x^2 = 24$$
$$x^2 = 4$$
$$x = \pm 2$$

The solution set is $\{\pm 2\}$.

45.
$$2t^2 = 7$$
$$t^2 = \frac{7}{2}$$
$$t = \pm \sqrt{\frac{7}{2}}$$
$$t = \pm \frac{\sqrt{14}}{2}$$

The solution set is $\{\pm \frac{\sqrt{14}}{2}\}$.

53.
$$(x-2)^2 = 9$$
$$x - 2 = \pm 3$$
$$x - 2 = -3 \text{ or } x - 2 = 3$$
$$x = -1 \text{ or } \quad x = 5$$

The solution set is $\{-1, 5\}$.

61.
$$(n-4)^2 = 5$$
$$n - 4 = \pm \sqrt{5}$$
$$n = 4 \pm \sqrt{5}$$

The solution set is $\{4 \pm \sqrt{5}\}$.

33.
$$2x^2 + 5kx - 3k^2 = 0$$
$$(2x - k)(x + 3k) = 0$$
$$2x - k = 0 \text{ or } x + 3k = 0$$
$$2x = k \text{ or } \quad x = -3k$$
$$x = \frac{k}{2} \text{ or } \quad x = -3k$$

The solution set is $\{-3k, \frac{k}{2}\}$.

41.
$$n^2 - 28 = 0$$
$$n^2 = 28$$
$$n = \pm \sqrt{28}$$
$$n = \pm 2\sqrt{7} \quad (\sqrt{28} = \sqrt{4}\sqrt{7} = 2\sqrt{7})$$

The solution set is $\{\pm 2\sqrt{7}\}$.

49.
$$10x^2 - 48 = 0$$
$$10x^2 = 48$$
$$5x^2 = 24$$
$$x^2 = \frac{24}{5}$$
$$x = \pm \sqrt{\frac{24}{5}}$$
$$x = \pm \frac{2\sqrt{30}}{5}$$

The solution set is $\{\pm \frac{2\sqrt{30}}{5}\}$.

57. The square of any number is non-negative. Thus, the solution set for $(x+6)^2 = -4$ is $\emptyset$.

65.
$$(3y-2)^2 = 27$$
$$3y - 2 = \pm \sqrt{27}$$
$$3y - 2 = \pm 3\sqrt{3}$$
$$3y = 2 \pm 3\sqrt{3}$$
$$y = \frac{2 \pm 3\sqrt{3}}{3}$$

The solution set is $\{\frac{2 \pm 3\sqrt{3}}{3}\}$.

69.
$$2(5x-2)^2 + 5 = 25$$
$$2(5x-2)^2 = 20$$
$$(5x-2)^2 = 10$$
$$5x-2 = \pm\sqrt{10}$$
$$5x = 2 \pm \sqrt{10}$$
$$x = \frac{2 \pm \sqrt{10}}{5}$$

The solution set is $\{\frac{2 \pm \sqrt{10}}{5}\}$.

73.
$$a^2 + b^2 = c^2$$
$$a^2 + (8)^2 = (12)^2$$
$$a^2 + 64 = 144$$
$$a^2 = 80$$
$$a = \sqrt{80} = 4\sqrt{5} \text{ inches}$$

77. If b = 6 inches, then a = 6 inches because it is an **isosceles right** triangle.
$$c^2 = a^2 + b^2$$
$$c^2 = (6)^2 + (6)^2$$
$$c^2 = 36 + 36$$
$$c^2 = 72$$
$$c = \sqrt{72} = 6\sqrt{2} \text{ inches}$$

81. The hypotenuse is twice as long as the side opposite the 30° angle. Therefore, c = 2(3) = 6 inches.
$$c^2 = a^2 + b^2$$
$$(6)^2 = (3)^2 + b^2$$
$$36 = 9 + b^2$$
$$27 = b^2$$
$$\sqrt{27} = b$$
$$b = 3\sqrt{3} \text{ inches}$$

85. The hypotenuse is twice as long as the side opposite the 30° angle. Therefore, c = 2a.
$$a^2 + b^2 = c^2$$
$$a^2 + (10)^2 = (2a)^2$$
$$a^2 + 100 = 4a^2$$
$$100 = 3a^2$$
$$\frac{100}{3} = a^2$$
$$\sqrt{\frac{100}{3}} = a$$
$$a = \frac{10\sqrt{3}}{3} \text{ feet}$$
and
$$c = 2\left(\frac{10\sqrt{3}}{3}\right) = \frac{20\sqrt{3}}{3} \text{ feet}$$

Problem Set 6.2

1.   <u>Factoring</u>   <u>Completing the Square</u>

$$x^2-4x-60 = 0$$
$$(x-10)(x+6) = 0$$
$$x-10 = 0 \text{ or } x+6 = 0$$
$$x = 10 \text{ or } x = -6$$

Completing the Square:
$$x^2-4x-60 = 0$$
$$x^2-4x = 60$$
$$x^2-4x+4 = 60+4$$
$$(x-2)^2 = 8^2$$
$$x-2 = \pm 8$$
$$x-2 = -8 \text{ or } x-2 = 8$$
$$x = -6 \text{ or } x = 10$$

The solution set is {-6 10}.

5.   <u>Factoring</u>   <u>Completing the Square</u>

$$x^2-5x-50 = 0$$
$$(x-10)(x+5) = 0$$
$$x-10 = 0 \text{ or } x+5 = 0$$
$$x = 10 \text{ or } x = -5$$

Completing the Square:
$$x^2-5x-50 = 0$$
$$x^2-5x = 50$$
$$x^2-5x+\frac{25}{4} = 50+\frac{25}{4}$$
$$\left(x-\frac{5}{2}\right)^2 = \left(\frac{15}{2}\right)^2$$
$$x-\frac{5}{2} = -\frac{15}{2} \text{ or } x-\frac{5}{2} = \frac{15}{2}$$
$$x = -5 \text{ or } x = 10$$

The solution set is {-5,10}.

9.   <u>Factoring</u>   <u>Completing the Square</u>

$$2n^2-n-15 = 0$$
$$(2n+5)(n-3) = 0$$
$$2n+5 = 0 \text{ or } n-3 = 0$$
$$2n = -5 \text{ or } n = 3$$
$$n = -\frac{5}{2} \text{ or } n = 3$$

Completing the Square:
$$2n^2-n-15 = 0$$
$$2n^2-n = 15$$
$$n^2-\frac{1}{2}n = \frac{15}{2}$$
$$n^2-\frac{1}{2}n+\frac{1}{16} = \frac{15}{2}+\frac{1}{16}$$
$$\left(n-\frac{1}{4}\right)^2 = \left(\frac{11}{4}\right)^2$$
$$n-\frac{1}{4} = -\frac{11}{4} \text{ or } n-\frac{1}{4} = \frac{11}{4}$$
$$n = -\frac{5}{2} \text{ or } n = 3$$

The solution set is $\{-\frac{5}{2}, 3\}$.

13.   Factoring   Completing the Square

$$n(n+6) = 160$$
$$n^2+6n-160 = 0$$
$$(n+16)(n-10) = 0$$
$$n+16 = 0 \quad \text{or } n-10 = 0$$
$$n = -16 \quad \text{or} \quad n = 10$$

The solution set is $\{-16, 10\}$.

$$n(n+6) = 160$$
$$n^2+6n = 160$$
$$n^2+6n+9 = 160+9$$
$$(n+3)^2 = (13)^2$$
$$n+3 = -13 \text{ or } n+3 = 13$$
$$n = -16 \text{ or} \quad n = 10$$

17.
$$x^2+6x-3 = 0$$
$$x^2+6x = 3$$
$$x^2+6x+9 = 3+9$$
$$(x+3)^2 = (\sqrt{12})^2 = (2\sqrt{3})^2$$
$$x+3 = \pm 2\sqrt{3}$$
$$x = -3 \pm 2\sqrt{3}$$

The solution set is $\{-3 \pm 2\sqrt{3}\}$.

21.
$$n^2-8n+4 = 0$$
$$n^2-8n = -4$$
$$n^2-8n+16 = -4+16$$
$$(n-4)^2 = (\sqrt{12})^2 = (2\sqrt{3})^2$$
$$n-4 = \pm 2\sqrt{3}$$
$$n = 4 \pm 2\sqrt{3}$$

The solution set is $\{4 \pm 2\sqrt{3}\}$.

25.
$$n^2+2n+6 = 0$$
$$n^2+2n = -6$$
$$n^2+2n+1 = -6+1$$
$$(n+1)^2 = -5$$

Since $(n+1)^2$ will always be non-negative, the solution set is $\emptyset$.

29.
$$x^2+5x+1 = 0$$
$$x^2+5x = -1$$
$$x^2+5x+\frac{25}{4} = -1+\frac{25}{4}$$
$$(x+\frac{5}{2})^2 = (\frac{\sqrt{21}}{2})^2$$
$$x+\frac{5}{2} = \pm\frac{\sqrt{21}}{2}$$
$$x = -\frac{5}{2} \pm \frac{\sqrt{21}}{2} = \frac{-5 \pm \sqrt{21}}{2}$$

The solution set is $\{\frac{-5 \pm \sqrt{21}}{2}\}$.

33.
$$2x^2+4x-3 = 0$$
$$2x^2+4x = 3$$
$$x^2+2x = \frac{3}{2}$$
$$x^2+2x+1 = \frac{3}{2}+1$$
$$(x+1)^2 = (\frac{\sqrt{10}}{2})^2 \qquad (\sqrt{\frac{5}{2}} = \sqrt{\frac{5}{2}\cdot\frac{2}{2}} = \sqrt{\frac{10}{4}} = \frac{\sqrt{10}}{2})$$
$$x+1 = \pm\frac{\sqrt{10}}{2}$$
$$x = -1 \pm \frac{\sqrt{10}}{2} = \frac{-2 \pm \sqrt{10}}{2}$$

The solution set is $\{\frac{-2 \pm \sqrt{10}}{2}\}$.

37. $3x^2+5x-1 = 0$

$$3x^2+5x = 1$$
$$x^2 +\frac{5}{3}x = \frac{1}{3}$$
$$x^2 +\frac{5}{3}x + \frac{25}{36} = \frac{1}{3}+\frac{25}{36}$$
$$(x +\frac{5}{6})^2 = (\frac{\sqrt{37}}{6})^2$$
$$x +\frac{5}{6} = \pm\frac{\sqrt{37}}{6}$$
$$x = -\frac{5}{6}\pm\frac{\sqrt{37}}{6} = \frac{-5\pm\sqrt{37}}{6}$$

The solution set is $\{\frac{-5\pm\sqrt{37}}{6}\}$.

41. $2n^2-8n = -3$

$$n^2-4n = -\frac{3}{2}$$
$$n^2-4n+4 = -\frac{3}{2}+4$$
$$(n-2)^2 = (\frac{\sqrt{10}}{2})^2$$
$$n-2 = \pm\frac{\sqrt{10}}{2}$$
$$n = \frac{2\pm\sqrt{10}}{2} = \frac{4\pm\sqrt{10}}{2}$$

The solution set is $\{\frac{4\pm\sqrt{10}}{2}\}$.

45. $(x+2)(x-7) = 10$

$$x^2-5x-14 = 10$$
$$x^2-5x-24 = 0$$
$$(x-8)(x+3) = 0$$
$$x-8 = 0 \text{ or } x+3 = 0$$
$$x = 8 \text{ or } x = -3$$

The solution set is $\{-3,8\}$.

49. $3n^2-6n-2 = 0$

$$3n^2-6n = 2$$
$$n^2-2n = \frac{2}{3}$$
$$n^2-2n+1 = \frac{2}{3}+1$$
$$(n-1)^2 = (\frac{\sqrt{15}}{3})^2$$
$$n-1 = \pm\frac{\sqrt{15}}{3}$$
$$n = 1\pm\frac{\sqrt{15}}{3} = \frac{3\pm\sqrt{15}}{3}$$

The solution set is $\{\frac{3\pm\sqrt{15}}{3}$.

53. $3x^2+29x = -66$

$$3x^2+29x+66 = 0$$
$$(3x+11)(x+6) = 0$$
$$3x+11 = 0 \text{ or } x+6 = 0$$
$$3x = -11 \text{ or } x = -6$$
$$x = -\frac{11}{3} \text{ or } x = -6$$

The solution set is $\{-6, -\frac{11}{3}\}$.

57. $x^2+12x = 4$

$$x^2+12x+36 = 4+36$$
$$(x+6)^2 = (2\sqrt{10})^2$$
$$x+6 = \pm 2\sqrt{10}$$
$$x = -6 \pm 2\sqrt{10}$$

The solution set is $\{-6 \pm 2\sqrt{10}\}$.

<u>Problem Set 6.3</u>

1. $b^2-4ac = (4)^2-4(1)(-21) = 16+84 = 100$

Since $b^2-4ac > 0$, the equation should have two real solutions.

$$x^2+4x-21 = 0$$
$$(x+7)(x-3) = 0$$
$$x+7 = 0 \quad \text{or} \quad x-3 = 0$$
$$x = -7 \quad \text{or} \quad x = 3$$

The solution set is $\{-7,3\}$.

5. $b^2-4ac = (-7)^2-4(1)(13) = 49-52 = -3$

Since $b^2-4ac < 0$, the equation has no real solutions. The solution set is $\emptyset$.

9. $b^2-4ac = (4)^2-4(3)(-2) = 16+24 = 40$

Since $b^2-4ac > 0$, the equation should have two real solutions.

$$3x^2+4x-2 = 0$$
$$x = \frac{-4 \pm \sqrt{16-4(3)(-2)}}{2(3)}$$
$$x = \frac{-4 \pm \sqrt{40}}{6}$$
$$x = \frac{-4 \pm 2\sqrt{10}}{6}$$
$$x = \frac{-2 \pm \sqrt{10}}{3}$$

The solution set is $\{\frac{-2 \pm \sqrt{10}}{3}\}$.

13. $n^2+5n-3 = 0$
$$n = \frac{-5 \pm \sqrt{25-4(1)(-3)}}{2}$$
$$n = \frac{-5 \pm \sqrt{37}}{2}$$

The solution set is $\{\frac{-5 \pm \sqrt{37}}{2}\}$.

17. $n^2+5n+8 = 0$
$$n = \frac{-5 \pm \sqrt{25-4(1)(8)}}{2}$$
$$n = \frac{-5 \pm \sqrt{-7}}{2}$$

Since $b^2-4ac < 0$, the equation has no real solutions. The solution set is $\emptyset$.

21.
$$-y^2 = -9y+5$$
$$-y^2+9y-5 = 0$$
$$y^2-9y+5 = 0$$
$$y = \frac{9 \pm \sqrt{81-4(1)(5)}}{2}$$
$$y = \frac{9 \pm \sqrt{61}}{2}$$

The solution set is $\{\frac{9 \pm \sqrt{61}}{2}\}$.

25.
$$4x^2+7x+2 = 0$$
$$x = \frac{-7 \pm \sqrt{49-4(4)(2)}}{2(4)}$$
$$x = \frac{-7 \pm \sqrt{17}}{8}$$

The solution set is $\{\frac{-7 \pm \sqrt{17}}{8}\}$.

29.
$$-2n^2+3n+5 = 0$$
$$2n^2-3n-5 = 0$$
$$n = \frac{3 \pm \sqrt{9-4(2)\cdot(-5)}}{2(2)}$$
$$n = \frac{3 \pm \sqrt{49}}{4} = \frac{3 \pm 7}{4}$$
$$n = \frac{3+7}{4} = \frac{5}{2} \text{ or } n = \frac{3-7}{4} = -1$$

The solution set is $\{-1, \frac{5}{2}\}$.

33.
$$36n^2-60n+25 = 0$$
$$n = \frac{60 \pm \sqrt{3600-4(36)(25)}}{2(36)}$$
$$n = \frac{60 \pm \sqrt{0}}{72}$$
$$n = \frac{60}{72} = \frac{5}{6}$$

The solution set is $\{\frac{5}{6}\}$.

37.
$$5x^2-13x = 0$$
$$x = \frac{13 \pm \sqrt{169-4(5)(0)}}{2(5)}$$
$$x = \frac{13 \pm \sqrt{169}}{10} = \frac{13 \pm 13}{10}$$
$$x = \frac{13+13}{10} = \frac{13}{5} \text{ or } x = \frac{13-13}{10} = 0$$

The solution set is $\{0, \frac{13}{5}\}$.

41.
$$6t^2+t-3 = 0$$
$$t = \frac{-1 \pm \sqrt{1-4(6)(-3)}}{2(6)}$$
$$t = \frac{-1 \pm \sqrt{73}}{12}$$

The solution set is $\{\frac{-1 \pm \sqrt{73}}{12}\}$.

45.
$$12x^2-73x+110 = 0$$
$$x = \frac{73 \pm \sqrt{5329-4(12)(110)}}{2(12)}$$
$$x = \frac{73 \pm \sqrt{49}}{24} = \frac{73 \pm 7}{24}$$
$$x = \frac{73-7}{24} = \frac{11}{4} \text{ or } x = \frac{73+7}{24} = \frac{10}{3}$$

The solution set is $\{\frac{11}{4}, \frac{10}{3}\}$.

49. $-6x^2+2x+1 = 0$

$6x^2-2x-1 = 0$

$$x = \frac{2 \pm \sqrt{4-4(6)(-1)}}{2(6)}$$

$$x = \frac{2 \pm \sqrt{28}}{12} = \frac{2 \pm 2\sqrt{7}}{12} = \frac{1 \pm \sqrt{7}}{6}$$

The solution set is $\{\frac{1 \pm \sqrt{7}}{6}\}$.

<u>Problem Set 6.4</u>

1. $x^2-4x-6 = 0$

$$x = \frac{4 \pm \sqrt{16-4(1)(-6)}}{2}$$

$$x = \frac{4 \pm \sqrt{40}}{2} = \frac{4 \pm 2\sqrt{10}}{2} = 2 \pm \sqrt{10}$$

The solution set is $\{2 \pm \sqrt{10}\}$.

9. $135+24n+n^2 = 0$

$n^2+24n+135 = 0$

$(n+15)(n+9) = 0$

$n+15 = 0$ or $n+9 = 0$

$n = -15$ or $n = -9$

The solution set is $\{-15,-9\}$.

17. $20y^2+17y-10 = 0$

$(5y-2)(4y+5) = 0$

$5y-2 = 0$ or $4y+5 = 0$

$5y = 2$ or $4y = -5$

$y = \frac{2}{5}$ or $y = -\frac{5}{4}$

The solution set is $\{-\frac{5}{4},\frac{2}{5}\}$.

5. $x^2-18x = 9$

$x^2-18x+81 = 9+81$

$(x-9)^2 = (3\sqrt{10})^2$

$x-9 = \pm 3\sqrt{10}$

$x = 9 \pm 3\sqrt{10}$

The solution set is $\{9 \pm 3\sqrt{10}\}$.

13. $2x^2-4x+7 = 0$

$$x = \frac{4 \pm \sqrt{16-4(2)(7)}}{2(2)}$$

$$x = \frac{4 \pm \sqrt{-40}}{2(2)}$$

Since $b^2-4ac < 0$, the equation has no real solutions. The solution set is $\emptyset$.

21. $n+\frac{3}{n} = \frac{19}{4}$, $n \neq 0$

$$4n(n+\frac{3}{n}) = 4n(\frac{19}{4})$$

$4n^2+12 = 19n$

$4n^2-19n+12 = 0$

$(4n-3)(n-4) = 0$

$4n-3 = 0$ or $n-4 = 0$

$4n = 3$ or $n = 4$

$n = \frac{3}{4}$ or $n = 4$

The solution set is $\{\frac{3}{4},4\}$.

25.

$$\frac{12}{x-3} + \frac{8}{x} = 14, \quad x \neq 3 \text{ and } x \neq 0$$

$$x(x-3)\left[\frac{12}{x-3} + \frac{8}{x}\right] = x(x-3)(14)$$

$$12x + 8(x-3) = 14x(x-3)$$

$$12x + 8x - 24 = 14x^2 - 42x$$

$$0 = 14x^2 - 62x + 24$$

$$0 = 7x^2 - 31x + 12$$

$$0 = (7x-3)(x-4)$$

$$7x - 3 = 0 \text{ or } x - 4 = 0$$

$$7x = 3 \text{ or } x = 4$$

$$x = \frac{3}{7} \text{ or } x = 4$$

The solution set is $\{\frac{3}{7}, 4\}$.

29.

$$\frac{6}{x} + \frac{40}{x+5} = 7, \quad x \neq 0 \text{ and } x \neq -5$$

$$x(x+5)\left[\frac{6}{x} + \frac{40}{x+5}\right] = x(x+5)(7)$$

$$6(x+5) + 40x = 7x^2 + 35x$$

$$6x + 30 + 4x = 7x^2 + 35x$$

$$46x + 30 = 7x^2 + 35x$$

$$0 = 7x^2 - 11x - 30$$

$$0 = (7x+10)(x-3)$$

$$7x + 10 = 0 \text{ or } x - 3 = 0$$

$$7x = -10 \text{ or } x = 3$$

$$x = -\frac{10}{7} \text{ or } x = 3$$

The solution set is $\{-\frac{10}{7}, 3\}$.

33.

$$x^4 - 18x^2 + 72 = 0$$

$$(x^2 - 12)(x^2 - 6) = 0$$

$$x^2 - 12 = 0 \text{ or } x^2 - 6 = 0$$

$$x^2 = 12 \text{ or } x^2 = 6$$

$$x = \pm\sqrt{12} \text{ or } x = \pm\sqrt{6}$$

$$x = \pm 2\sqrt{3} \text{ or } x = \pm\sqrt{6}$$

The solution set is $\{\pm\sqrt{6}, \pm 2\sqrt{3}\}$.

37.

$$3x^4 - 2x^2 - 5 = 0$$

$$(3x^2 - 5)(x^2 + 1) = 0$$

$$3x^2 - 5 = 0 \text{ or } x^2 + 1 = 0$$

$$3x^2 = 5 \text{ or } x^2 = -1$$

$$x^2 = \frac{5}{3} \text{ or } x^2 = -1$$

$$x = \pm\sqrt{\frac{5}{3}} = \pm\frac{\sqrt{15}}{3} \text{ or } x^2 = -1$$

The equation $x^2 = -1$ produces no real number solutions. The solution set of the given equation is

$$\{\pm\frac{\sqrt{15}}{3}\}.$$

41. Let n and n+1 represent the two consecutive whole numbers.

$$n^2 + (n+1)^2 = 145$$

$$n^2 + n^2 + 2n + 1 = 145$$

$$2n^2 + 2n - 144 = 0$$

$$n^2 + n - 72 = 0$$

$$(n+9)(n-8) = 0$$

$$n + 9 = 0 \text{ or } n - 8 = 0$$

$$n = -9 \text{ or } n = 8$$

The solution of −9 must be discarded since the problem pertains to <u>whole</u> <u>numbers</u>. Thus, the whole numbers are 8 and 8+1 = 9.

45. Let n and 10−n represent the two numbers.

$$n(10-n) = 22$$

$$10n - n^2 = 22$$

$$0 = n^2 - 10n + 22$$

$$n = \frac{10 \pm \sqrt{100-88}}{2}$$

$$= \frac{10 \pm \sqrt{12}}{2} = \frac{10 \pm 2\sqrt{3}}{2}$$

$$= 5 \pm \sqrt{3}$$

The numbers are $5 + \sqrt{3}$ and $5 - \sqrt{3}$.

49.

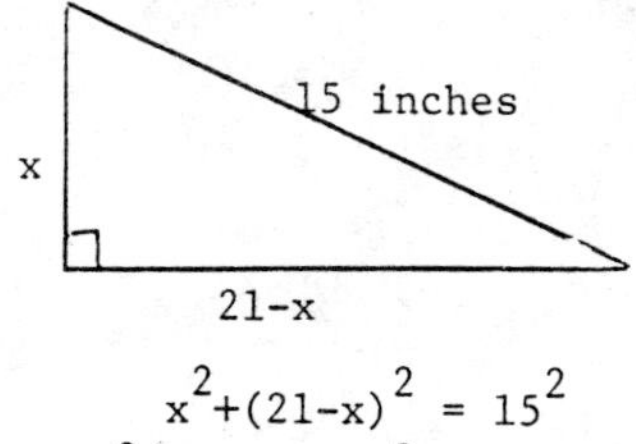

$$x^2+(21-x)^2 = 15^2$$
$$x^2+441-42x+x^2 = 225$$
$$2x^2-42x+216 = 0$$
$$x^2-21x+108 = 0$$
$$(x-9)(x-12) = 0$$
$$x-9 = 0 \text{ or } x-12 = 0$$
$$x = 9 \text{ or } \quad x = 12$$

If x = 9, then 21-x = 21-9 = 12 and if x = 12, then 21-x = 21-12 = 9. The legs are 9 inches and 12 inches long.

53. Let w represent the width of the rectangle. Then $\frac{44-2w}{2} = 22-w$ represents the length.

$$w(22-w) = 112$$
$$22w-w^2 = 112$$
$$0 = w^2-22w+112$$
$$0 = (w-8)(w-14)$$
$$w-8 = 0 \text{ or } w-14 = 0$$
$$w = 8 \text{ or } \quad w = 14$$

If w = 8, then 22-w = 22-8 = 14.
If w = 14, then 22-w = 22-14 = 8.
The rectangle is 8 inches by 14 inches.

57.

	d	r	t
first part of trip	330	x	$\frac{330}{x}$
last part of trip	240	x+5	$\frac{240}{x+5}$

Since the entire trip took 10 hours we can set up and solve the following equation.

$$\frac{330}{x} + \frac{240}{x+5} = 10$$
$$330(x+5)+240x = 10x(x+5)$$
$$330x+1650+240x = 10x^2+50x$$
$$0 = 10x^2-520x-1650$$
$$0 = x^2-52x-165$$
$$0 = (x-55)(x+3)$$
$$x-55 = 0 \text{ or } x+3 = 0$$
$$x = 55 \text{ or } \quad x = -3$$

The negative solution must be discarded; so Andy traveled at 55 miles per hour for the first part of the trip.

61. Let h be the number of hours he expected the job to take. Then h+6 represents the number of hours it actually took.

$$\frac{360}{h+6} = \frac{360}{h} - 2$$
$$360h = 360(h+6)-2h(h+6)$$
$$360h = 360h+2160-2h^2-12h$$
$$2h^2+12h-2160 = 0$$
$$h^2+6h-1080 = 0$$
$$(h+36((h-30) = 0$$
$$h+36 = 0 \text{ or } h-30 = 0$$
$$h = -36 \text{ or } \quad h = 30$$

The negative solution must be discarded.
Thus, he expected it to take 30 hours.

65. Let x represent the number of
shares that he bought. Then x-20
represents the number of shares
that he sold.

$$\frac{800}{x-20} = \frac{720}{x} + 8$$

$$800x = 720(x-20)+8x(x-20)$$

$$800x = 720x-14400+8x^2-160x$$

$$0 = 8x^2-240x-14400$$

$$0 = x^2-30x-1800$$

$$0 = (x-60)(x+30)$$

$$x-60 = 0 \quad \text{or} \quad x+30 = 0$$

$$x = 60 \text{ or} \quad x = -30$$

The negative solution must be discarded. Therefore, he sold x-20 =

$60-20 = 40$ shares at $\frac{\$800}{40} = \$20$ per
share.

69.

$$A = P(1+r)^t$$

$$594.05 = 500(1+r)^2$$

$$1.1881 = (1+r)^2$$

$$\sqrt{1.1881} = 1+r$$

$$1.09 = 1+r$$

$$.09 = r$$

The rate of interest is 9%.

Problem Set 6.5

1.

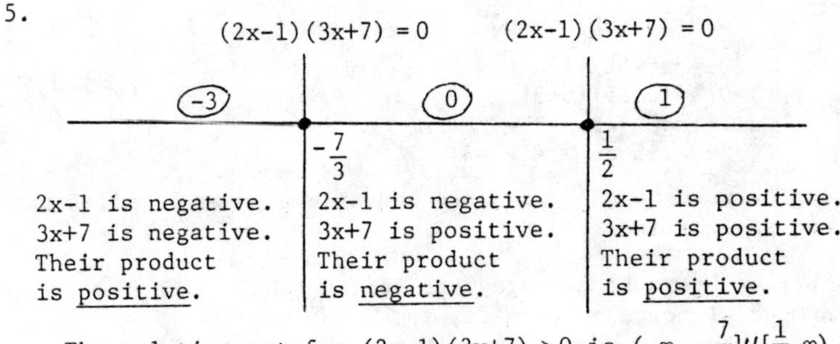

$$(x+2)(x-1) = 0 \qquad (x+2)(x-1) = 0$$

x+2 is negative.	x+2 is positive.	x+2 is positive.
x-1 is negative.	x-1 is negative.	x-1 is positive.
Their product	Their product	Their product
is positive.	is negative.	is positive.

The solution set for $(x+2)(x-1) > 0$ is $(-\infty,-2)\cup(1,\infty)$.

5.

$$(2x-1)(3x+7) = 0 \qquad (2x-1)(3x+7) = 0$$

2x-1 is negative.	2x-1 is negative.	2x-1 is positive.
3x+7 is negative.	3x+7 is positive.	3x+7 is positive.
Their product	Their product	Their product
is positive.	is negative.	is positive.

The solution set for $(2x-1)(3x+7) \geq 0$ is $(-\infty, -\frac{7}{3}]\cup[\frac{1}{2},\infty)$.

9.

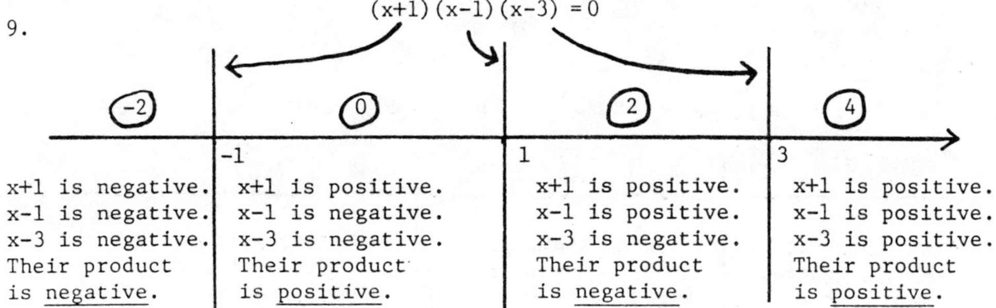

$$(x+1)(x-1)(x-3) = 0$$

-2	0	2	4
x+1 is negative. x-1 is negative. x-3 is negative. Their product is <u>negative</u>.	x+1 is positive. x-1 is negative. x-3 is negative. Their product is <u>positive</u>.	x+1 is positive. x-1 is positive. x-3 is negative. Their product is <u>negative</u>.	x+1 is positive. x-1 is positive. x-3 is positive. Their product is <u>positive</u>.

The solution set for $(x+1)(x-1)(x-3) > 0$ is $(-1,1) \cup (3,\infty)$.

13.

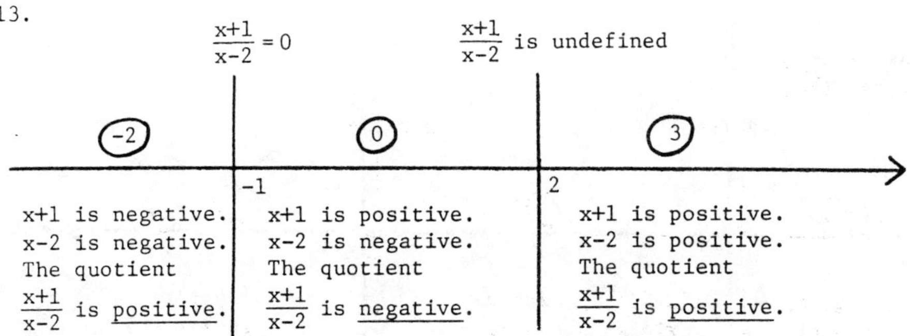

$$\frac{x+1}{x-2} = 0 \qquad\qquad \frac{x+1}{x-2} \text{ is undefined}$$

-2	0	3
x+1 is negative. x-2 is negative. The quotient $\frac{x+1}{x-2}$ is <u>positive</u>.	x+1 is positive. x-2 is negative. The quotient $\frac{x+1}{x-2}$ is <u>negative</u>.	x+1 is positive. x-2 is positive. The quotient $\frac{x+1}{x-2}$ is <u>positive</u>.

The solution set for $\frac{x+1}{x-2} > 0$ is $(-\infty,-1) \cup (2,\infty)$.

17.

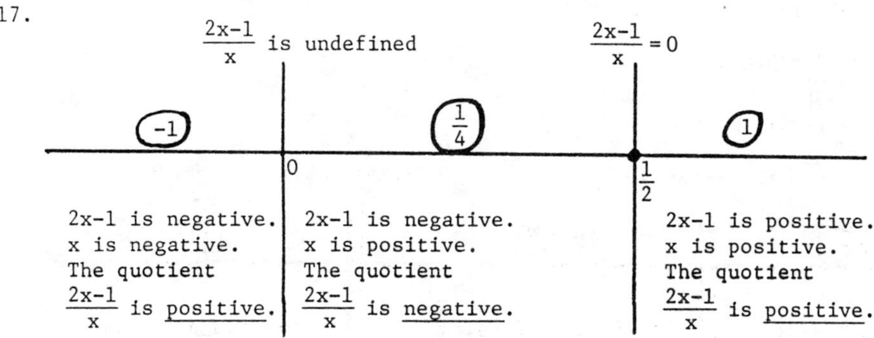

$$\frac{2x-1}{x} \text{ is undefined} \qquad\qquad \frac{2x-1}{x} = 0$$

-1	$\frac{1}{4}$	1
2x-1 is negative. x is negative. The quotient $\frac{2x-1}{x}$ is <u>positive</u>.	2x-1 is negative. x is positive. The quotient $\frac{2x-1}{x}$ is <u>negative</u>.	2x-1 is positive. x is positive. The quotient $\frac{2x-1}{x}$ is <u>positive</u>.

The solution set for $\frac{2x-1}{x} \geq 0$ is $(-\infty,0) \cup [\frac{1}{2},\infty)$.

21. $x^2 + 2x - 35 < 0$
$(x+7)(x-5) < 0$

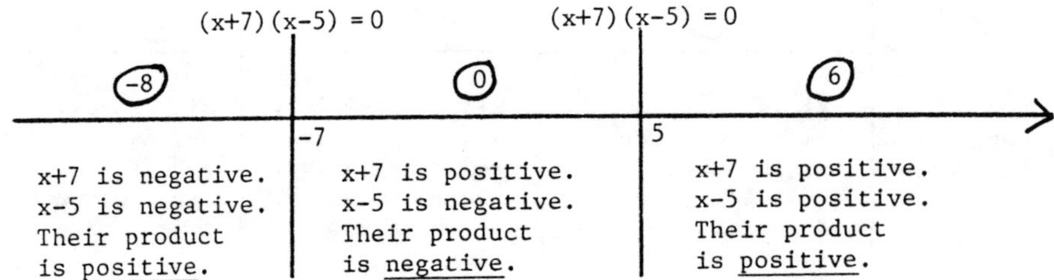

The solution set is $(-7, 5)$.

25. $3x^2 + 13x - 10 \leq 0$
$(3x-2)(x+5) \leq 0$

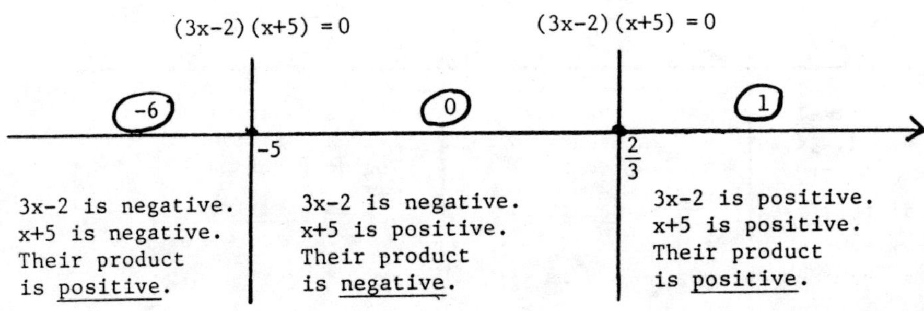

The solution set is $[-5, \frac{2}{3}]$.

29. $x(5x-36) > 32$
$5x^2 - 36x - 32 > 0$
$(5x+4)(x-8) > 0$

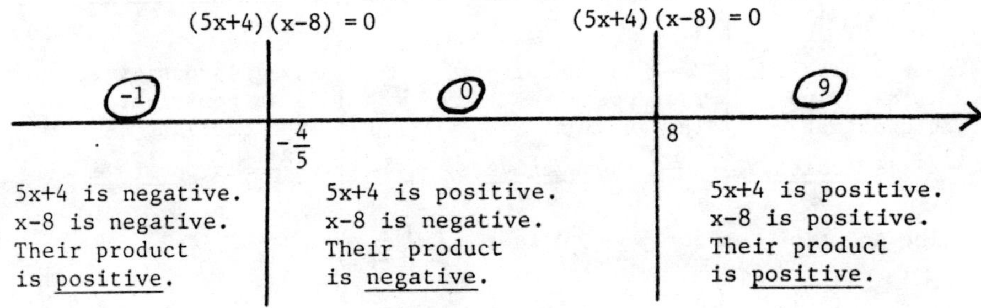

The solution set is $(-\infty, -\frac{4}{5}) \cup (8, \infty)$.

33. $$4x^2+20x+25 < 0$$
$$(2x+5)(2x+5) < 0$$
$$(2x+5)^2 < 0$$

The quantity $(2x+5)^2$ equals zero when $x = -\frac{5}{2}$ but is positive for all other values of x. Thus, the solution set is $\{-\frac{5}{2}\}$.

37. $$\frac{2x}{x+3} > 4$$
$$\frac{2x}{x+3} - 4 > 0$$
$$\frac{2x-4(x+3)}{x+3} > 0$$
$$\frac{2x-4x-12}{x+3} > 0$$
$$\frac{-2x-12}{x+3} > 0$$

$\dfrac{-2x-12}{x+3} = 0 \qquad \dfrac{-2x-12}{x+3}$ is undefined

-7	-4	0

-6 $\qquad$ -3

-2x-12 is positive.   -2x-12 is negative.   -2x-12 is negative.
x+3 is negative.   x+3 is negative.   x+3 is positive.
The quotient   The quotient   The quotient
$\dfrac{-2x-12}{x+3}$ is negative. $\dfrac{-2x-12}{x+3}$ is positive. $\dfrac{-2x-12}{x+3}$ is negative.

The solution set is $(-6,-3)$.

41. $$\frac{x+2}{x-3} > -2$$
$$\frac{x+2}{x-3} + 2 > 0$$
$$\frac{x+2+2(x-3)}{x-3} > 0$$
$$\frac{x+2+2x-6}{x-3} > 0$$
$$\frac{3x-4}{x-3} > 0$$

$\dfrac{3x-4}{x-3} > 0 \qquad \dfrac{3x-4}{x-3} = 0 \qquad \dfrac{3x-4}{x-3}$ is undefined

1	2	4

$\frac{4}{3}$ $\qquad$ 3

3x-4 is negative.   3x-4 is positive.   3x-4 is positive.
x-3 is negative.   x-3 is negative.   x-3 is positive.
The quotient   The quotient   The quotient
$\dfrac{3x-4}{x-3}$ is positive. $\dfrac{3x-4}{x-3}$ is negative. $\dfrac{3x-4}{x-3}$ is positive.

The solution set is $(-\infty,\frac{4}{3}) \cup (3,\infty)$.

45. $\dfrac{x+1}{x-2} < 1$

$\dfrac{x+1}{x-2} - 1 < 0$

$\dfrac{x+1-1(x-2)}{x-2} < 0$

$\dfrac{x+1-x+2}{x-2} < 0$

$\dfrac{3}{x-2} < 0$

The numerator, 3, is positive. Thus, x-2 must be negative so that the quotient is negative.

$$x-2 < 0$$
$$x < 2$$

The solution set is $(-\infty, 2)$.

Problem Set 6.6

1. This statement is <u>false</u> because a number such as 3+2i is complex but not a real number.

5. This statement is <u>true</u> because (a+bi)+(c+di) = (a+c)+(b+d)i which is a complex number.

9. $(6+3i)+(4+5i) = (6+4)+(3+5)i = 10+8i$

13. $(3+2i)-(5+7i) = (3+2i)+(-5-7i) = -2-5i$

17. $(-3-10i)+(2-13i) = (-3+2)+(-10-13)i = -1-23i$

21. $(-1-i)-(-2-4i) = (-1-i)+(2+4i) = 1+3i$

25. $\left(-\dfrac{5}{9}+\dfrac{3}{5}i\right)-\left(\dfrac{4}{3}-\dfrac{1}{6}i\right) = \left(-\dfrac{5}{9}+\dfrac{3}{5}i\right)+\left(-\dfrac{4}{3}+\dfrac{1}{6}i\right) = \left(-\dfrac{5}{9}-\dfrac{4}{3}\right)+\left(\dfrac{3}{5}+\dfrac{1}{6}\right)i = -\dfrac{17}{9}+\dfrac{23}{30}i$

29. $\sqrt{-14} = i\sqrt{14}$
    33. $\sqrt{-18} = i\sqrt{18} = i\sqrt{9}\sqrt{2} = 3i\sqrt{2}$

37. $3\sqrt{-28} = 3i\sqrt{28} = 3i\sqrt{4}\sqrt{7} = 6i\sqrt{7}$
    41. $12\sqrt{-90} = 12i\sqrt{90} = 12i\sqrt{9}\sqrt{10} = 36i\sqrt{10}$

45. $\sqrt{-3}\sqrt{-5} = (i\sqrt{3})(i\sqrt{5}) = i^2\sqrt{15} = -\sqrt{15}$

49. $\sqrt{-15}\sqrt{-5} = (i\sqrt{15})(i\sqrt{5}) = i^2\sqrt{75} = (-1)\sqrt{25}\sqrt{3} = -5\sqrt{3}$

53. $\sqrt{6}\sqrt{-8} = (\sqrt{6})(i\sqrt{8}) = i\sqrt{48} = i\sqrt{16}\sqrt{3} = 4i\sqrt{3}$

57. $\dfrac{\sqrt{-56}}{\sqrt{-7}} = \dfrac{i\sqrt{56}}{i\sqrt{7}} = \sqrt{\dfrac{56}{7}} = \sqrt{8} = \sqrt{4}\sqrt{2} = 2\sqrt{2}$

61. $(5i)(4i) = 20i^2 = 20(-1) = -20 = -20+0i$

65. $3i(2-5i) = 3i(2) - 3i(5i) = 6i - 15i^2 = 6i - 15(-1) = 15+6i$

69. $(3+2i)(5+4i) = 3(5+4i)+2i(5+4i) = 15+12i+10i+8i^2 = 15+22i+8(-1) = 7+22i$

73. $(-3-2i)(5+6i) = -3(5+6i)-2i(5+6i) = -15-18i-10i-12i^2 = -15-28i-12(-1)$

$$= -3-28i$$

77. $(4+5i)^2 = (4)^2+2(4)(5i)+(5i)^2 = 16+40i+25i^2 = 16+40i+25(-1) = -9+40i$

81. $(6+7i)(6-7i) = (6)^2-(7i)^2 = 36-49i^2 = 36-49(-1) = 85 = 85+0i$

85. $\dfrac{3i}{2+4i} = \dfrac{3i}{2+4i} \cdot \dfrac{2-4i}{2-4i} = \dfrac{3i(2-4i)}{4-16i^2} = \dfrac{6i-12i^2}{4-16(-1)} = \dfrac{6i-12(-1)}{4+16} = \dfrac{12+6i}{20}$

$$= \dfrac{12}{20} + \dfrac{6}{20}i = \dfrac{3}{5} + \dfrac{3}{10}i$$

89. $\dfrac{-2+6i}{3i} = \dfrac{-2+6i}{3i} \cdot \dfrac{i}{i} = \dfrac{-2i+6i^2}{3i^2} = \dfrac{-6-2i}{-3} = 2 + \dfrac{2}{3}i$

93. $\dfrac{2+6i}{1+7i} = \dfrac{2+6i}{1+7i} \cdot \dfrac{1-7i}{1-7i} = \dfrac{2-14i+6i-42i^2}{1-49i^2} = \dfrac{2-8i+42}{1+49} = \dfrac{44-8i}{50} = \dfrac{22}{25} - \dfrac{4}{25}i$

97. $\dfrac{-2+7i}{-1+i} \cdot \dfrac{-1-i}{-1-i} = \dfrac{2+2i-7i-7i^2}{1-i^2} = \dfrac{2-5i-7(-1)}{1-(-1)} = \dfrac{9-5i}{2} = \dfrac{9}{2} - \dfrac{5}{2}i$

Problem Set 6.7

1. $x^2 = -64$

$\quad x = \pm\sqrt{-64} = \pm i\sqrt{64} = \pm 8i$

The solution set is $\{\pm 8i\}$.

5. $(x-1)^2 = -7$

$\quad x-1 = \pm\sqrt{-7} = \pm i\sqrt{7}$

$\quad x = 1 \pm i\sqrt{7}$

The solution set is $\{1 \pm i\sqrt{7}\}$.

9. $(2x+3)^2 = 1$

$\quad 2x+3 = \pm\sqrt{1} = \pm 1$

$2x+3 = -1$ or $2x+3 = 1$

$\quad 2x = -4$ or $\quad 2x = -2$

$\quad x = -2$ or $\quad\quad x = -1$

The solution set is $\{-2,-1\}$.

13. $x^2-4x = 20$

$\quad x^2-4x+4 = -20+4$

$\quad (x-2)^2 = -16$

$\quad\quad x-2 = \pm\sqrt{-16} = \pm i\sqrt{16} = \pm 4i$

$\quad\quad\quad x = 2 \pm 4i$

The solution set is $\{2 \pm 4i\}$.

17. $n^2 = -4n-1$

$n^2+4n+1 = 0$

$\quad n = \dfrac{-4 \pm \sqrt{16-4(1)(1)}}{2}$

$\quad n = \dfrac{-4 \pm \sqrt{12}}{2} = \dfrac{-4 \pm 2\sqrt{3}}{2}$

$\quad\quad = -2 \pm \sqrt{3}$

The solution set is $\{-2 \pm \sqrt{3}\}$.

21. $3x^2-2x+5 = 0$

$\quad x = \dfrac{2 \pm \sqrt{4-4(3)(5)}}{2(3)}$

$\quad x = \dfrac{2 \pm \sqrt{-56}}{6} = \dfrac{2 \pm i\sqrt{56}}{6}$

$\quad x = \dfrac{2 \pm 2i\sqrt{14}}{6} = \dfrac{1 \pm i\sqrt{14}}{3}$

The solution set is $\{\dfrac{1 \pm i\sqrt{14}}{3}\}$.

25. $5x^2-4x+4 = 0$

$\quad x = \dfrac{4 \pm \sqrt{16-4(5)(4)}}{2(5)}$

$\quad x = \dfrac{4 \pm \sqrt{-64}}{10} = \dfrac{4 \pm 8i}{10} = \dfrac{2 \pm 4i}{5}$

The solution set is $\{\dfrac{2 \pm 4i}{5}\}$.

29. $5x^2-2x+3 = 0$

$\quad x = \dfrac{2 \pm \sqrt{4-4(5)(3)}}{2(5)}$

$\quad x = \dfrac{2 \pm \sqrt{-56}}{10} = \dfrac{2 \pm i\sqrt{56}}{10}$

$\quad x = \dfrac{2 \pm 2i\sqrt{14}}{10} = \dfrac{1 \pm i\sqrt{14}}{5}$

The solution set is $\{\dfrac{1 \pm i\sqrt{14}}{5}\}$.

33. $x^2-8x+25 = 0$

$$x = \frac{8 \pm \sqrt{64-4(1)(25)}}{2}$$

$$x = \frac{8 \pm \sqrt{-36}}{2} = \frac{8 \pm 6i}{2} = 4 \pm 3i$$

The solution set is $\{4 \pm 3i\}$.

37. $3x^2+6x+4 = 0$

$$x = \frac{-6 \pm \sqrt{36-4(3)(4)}}{2(3)}$$

$$x = \frac{-6 \pm \sqrt{-12}}{6} = \frac{-6 \pm 2i\sqrt{3}}{6}$$

$$x = \frac{-3 \pm i\sqrt{3}}{3}$$

The solution set is $\{\frac{-3 \pm i\sqrt{3}}{3}\}$.

41. $b^2-4ac = (6)^2-4(1)(-7) = 36+28 = 64$

Since $b^2-4ac > 0$, the equation has two unequal real solutions.

45. $b^2-4ac = (5)^2-4(2)(7) = 25-56 = -31$

Since $b^2-4ac < 0$, the equation has two complex but nonreal solutions.

49. $6x(x-2) = -13$

$6x^2-12x+13 = 0$

$b^2-4ac = (-12)^2-4(6)(13) = 144-312 = -168$

Since $b^2-4ac < 0$, the equation has two complex but nonreal solutions.

53. $b^2-4ac = (-k)^2-4(3)(-2) = k^2+24$

Since k^2+24 will always be positive, any real value of k will produce real solutions.

Chapter 7

Problem Set 7.1

The graphs in this problem set are to be determined by following the suggestions offered at the end of Section 7.1 in the text. Primarily, you need to plot a sufficient number of points to determine the shape of the graph. You may need to plot even more points than what we have indicated in the answer section.

Problem Set 7.2

The graphs of this section are all straight lines. As suggested in the text, all we need to do is to plot two points (a third point can be found as a check point) and draw the line determined by the two points. Usually the intercepts can be easily determined and used as the two points. Don't forget that to find the x-intercept, let $y = 0$ and solve for x. Likewise, to find the y-intercept, let $x = 0$ and solve for y. I will illustrate the general approach with Problems 1 and 21.

1. $x+2y = 4$

Let $x = 0$; then $0+2y = 4$
$$2y = 4$$
$$y = 2.$$

So, the point $(0,2)$ is on the line.

Let $y = 0$; then $x+2(0) = 4$
$$x = 4.$$

So, the point $(4,0)$ is also on the line.

Draw the line determined by the two points $(0,2)$ and $(4,0)$.

Now let's find one more solution to use as a check.

Let $x = 2$; then $2+2y = 4$
$$2y = 2$$
$$y = 1.$$

So, the point $(2,1)$ should also be on the line.

If the check point does not appear to be on the line, then you should go back and check your work when finding the intercepts.

21. $y = 3x$

We should recognize that this line contains the origin; that is to say, the ordered pair $(0,0)$ satisfies the equation. So we should use the origin and two other points to graph the line. A small table of values can be used.

x	y
0	0
1	3
2	6

Thus, the points $(0,0),(1,3)$, and $(2,6)$ are on the line.

Problem Set 7.3

<u>The inequalities in Problems 1-18, inclusive, can be graphed by following the suggestions offered in the text. We shall illustrate this procedure with Problem 1.</u>

1. $x-y > 2$

    Step 1:   Graph $x-y = 2$ as a dashed line since equality is not included in the inequality statement.

    Step 2:   Choose the origin as a test point.

               $x-y > 2$ becomes $0-0 > 2$, which is a false statement.

    Step 3:   Since the test point did not satisfy the inequality, the part of the plane on the opposite side of the line from the origin (test point) should be shaded.

21. The statement $x > 1$ <u>and</u> $y < 3$ means that all points with x-coordinates larger than 1 and y-coordinates less than 3 are to be included. Thus, the lines $x = 1$ and $y = 3$ should be drawn as dashed lines. Then the region to the right of $x = 1$ and below $y = 3$ should be shaded.

Problem Set 7.4

1. $d = \sqrt{(x_2-x_1)^2+(y_2-y_1)^2} = \sqrt{[7-(-2)]^2+[11-(-1)]^2}$

$$= \sqrt{9^2+12^2} = \sqrt{81+144} = \sqrt{225} = 15$$

(Remember that the points can be labeled P_1 and P_2 in either order.)

5. $d = \sqrt{(x_2-x_1)^2+(y_2-y_1)^2} = \sqrt{(9-6)^2+[-7-(-4)]^2}$

$$= \sqrt{3^2+(-3)^2} = \sqrt{9+9} = \sqrt{18} = \sqrt{9}\sqrt{2} = 3\sqrt{2}$$

9. $d = \sqrt{(x_2-x_1)^2+(y_2-y_1)^2} = \sqrt{(-5-1)^2+[-6-(-6)]^2}$

$$= \sqrt{(-6)^2+(0)^2} = \sqrt{36} = 6$$

13. Let's label the points $A(-3,1)$, $B(5,7)$, and $C(8,3)$. Now we can find the lengths of the line segments $\overline{AB}$, $\overline{AC}$, and $\overline{BC}$.

$$AB = \sqrt{[5-(-3)]^2+(7-1)^2} = \sqrt{64+36} = \sqrt{100} = 10$$

$$AC = \sqrt{[8-(-3)]^2+(3-1)^2} = \sqrt{121+4} = \sqrt{125} = 5\sqrt{5}$$

$$BC = \sqrt{(8-5)^2+(3-7)^2} = \sqrt{9+16} = \sqrt{25} = 5$$

$$(AB)^2+(BC)^2 = 10^2+5^2 = 125 = (AC)^2$$

Therefore, it is a right triangle.

17. $m = \dfrac{y_2-y_1}{x_2-x_1} = \dfrac{6-2}{4-1} = \dfrac{4}{3}$
               21. $m = \dfrac{y_2-y_1}{x_2-x_1} = \dfrac{-2-6}{6-2} = \dfrac{-8}{4} = -2$

25. $\quad m = \dfrac{y_2 - y_1}{x_2 - x_1} = \dfrac{-4-(-4)}{2-(-2)} = \dfrac{0}{4} = 0$

29. Set the slope determined by $(-2,4)$ and $(x,6)$ equal to $\dfrac{2}{9}$ and solve for x.

$$\frac{6-4}{x-(-2)} = \frac{2}{9}$$

$$\frac{2}{x+2} = \frac{2}{9}$$

$$2(x+2) = 2(9)$$
$$2x+4 = 18$$
$$2x = 14$$
$$x = 7$$

33. and 37. These answers will vary. Points can be found by moving from the given point according to the given slope, keeping in mind that slope means

$$\frac{\text{change in y}}{\text{change in x}} \, .$$

Therefore, for Problem 33 where the slope is $\dfrac{1}{2}$ and the given point is $(2,5)$ we can find another point by moving up 1 unit and to the right 2 units. This would determine the point $(4,6)$.

41. Any two points can be used to determine the slope of a line. We will use the points determined by the intercepts.

Let $x = 0$; then $2(0)+3y = 6$
$$3y = 6$$
$$y = 2.$$

Thus, the point $(0,2)$ is on the line.

Let $y = 0$; then $2x+3(0) = 6$
$$2x = 6$$
$$x = 3.$$

Thus, the point $(3,0)$ is on the line.

Now we can use the two points $(0,2)$ and $(3,0)$ to determine the slope.

$$m = \frac{y_2 - y_1}{x_2 - x_1} = \frac{0-2}{3-0} = \frac{-2}{3} = -\frac{2}{3}$$

45. Let $x = 0$; then $4(0)-7y = 12$
$$-7y = 12$$
$$y = -\frac{12}{7}.$$

Let $y = 0$; then $4x-7(0) = 12$
$$4x = 12$$
$$x = 3.$$

The points $\left(0, -\dfrac{12}{7}\right)$ and $(3,0)$ can be used to determine the slope.

$$m = \frac{0-\left(-\dfrac{12}{7}\right)}{3-0} = \frac{\dfrac{12}{7}}{3} = \frac{12}{7} \cdot \frac{1}{3} = \frac{4}{7}$$

49. Let x = 0; then y = -5(0) = 0.

   Let x = 1; then y = -5(1) = -5.

   The points (0,0) and (1,-5) can be used to determine the slope.

   $$m = \frac{-5-0}{1-0} = \frac{-5}{1} = -5$$

Problem Set 7.5

Problems 1-8 can be done by either using the general approach illustrated in Example 1 of this section or by using the point-slope form of a straight line. We will use the general approach for Problem 1 and the point-slope form for Problem 5.

1. Choose some point (x,y) on the line and set the slope determined by that point and the given point $(3,5)$ equal to the given slope $\frac{1}{2}$.

$$\frac{y-5}{x-3} = \frac{1}{2}$$
$$1(x-3) = 2(y-5)$$
$$x-3 = 2y-10$$
$$x-2y = -7$$

5. Substitute the given ordered pair $(-1,-3)$ and the given slope, $-\frac{3}{4}$, into the point-slope form.

$$y-y_1 = m(x-x_1)$$
$$y-(-3) = -\frac{3}{4}(x-(-1))$$
$$y+3 = -\frac{3}{4}(x+1)$$
$$4y+12 = -3x-3$$
$$3x+4y = -15$$

Problems 9-18 can be done by first finding the slope using the two given points, and then using either approach from Problems 1-8.

9. The slope determined by $(2,1)$ and $(6,5)$ is

$$m = \frac{5-1}{6-2} = \frac{4}{4} = 1.$$

Now we can use either point and the slope in the point-slope form. We will use the point $(2,1)$.

$$y-y_1 = m(x-x_1)$$
$$y-1 = 1(x-2)$$
$$y-1 = x-2$$
$$1 = x-y$$

13. The slope determined by $(-3,2)$ and $(4,1)$ is

$$m = \frac{1-2}{4-(-3)} = \frac{-1}{7} = -\frac{1}{7}.$$

Now we can use either of the two points and the slope in the point-slope form. We will use the point $(4,1)$.

$$y-y_1 = m(x-x_1)$$
$$y-1 = -\frac{1}{7}(x-4)$$
$$7y-7 = -x+4$$
$$x+7y = 11$$

17. The slope determined by $(0,0)$ and $(5,7)$ is
$$m = \frac{7-0}{5-0} = \frac{7}{5}.$$

   Now we can use either of the two points and the slope in the point-slope form. We will use the point $(0,0)$.
$$y-y_1 = m(x-x_1)$$
$$y-0 = \frac{7}{5}(x-0)$$
$$y = \frac{7}{5}x$$
$$5y = 7x$$
$$0 = 7x-5y$$

21. Substitute 2 for m and -3 for b in the slope-intercept form.
$$y = mx+b$$
$$y = 2x-3$$

25. Substitute 0 for m and -4 for b in the slope-intercept form.
$$y = mx+b$$
$$y = 0(x)-4$$
$$y = -4$$

29. We can use the point $(-3,0)$ and the slope $-\frac{5}{8}$ in the point-slope form.
$$y-y_1 = m(x-x_1)$$
$$y-0 = -\frac{5}{8}(x-(-3))$$
$$y = -\frac{5}{8}(x+3)$$
$$8y = -5x-15$$
$$5x+8y = -15$$

33. Any horizontal line has an equation of the form $y = k$. Since this line contains the point $(5,6)$, its equation is $y = 6$ which can be written in standard form as $0(x)+y = 6$.

37. Since the line is to be parallel to $4x-7y = 3$, it must have the same slope. We can find that slope by changing $4x-7y = 3$ to slope-intercept form.
$$4x-7y = 3$$
$$-7y = -4x+3$$
$$y = \frac{4}{7}x - \frac{3}{7}$$
$$\uparrow$$
$$m = \frac{4}{7}$$

   Now we can use $m = \frac{4}{7}$ and the origin $(0,0)$ in the point-slope form.

$$y - y_1 = m(x - x_1)$$

$$y - 0 = \frac{4}{7}(x - 0)$$

$$y = \frac{4}{7}x$$

$$7y = 4x$$

$$0 = 4x - 7y$$

41. First, let's find the slope of the given line by changing to slope-intercept form.

$$-2x + 3y = 8$$

$$3y = 2x + 8$$

$$y = \frac{2}{3}x + \frac{8}{3}$$

The slope of the given line is $\frac{2}{3}$ and therefore the slope of any line perpendicular to it is $-\frac{3}{2}$. Now we can use the origin $(0,0)$ and the slope $-\frac{3}{2}$ in the point-slope form.

$$y - y_1 = m(x - x_1)$$

$$y - 0 = -\frac{3}{2}(x - 0)$$

$$y = -\frac{3}{2}x$$

$$2y = -3x$$

$$3x + 2y = 0$$

Problem Set 7.6

[Remember that the term "basic parabola" refers to the graph of $y = x^2$.]

1. $y = x^2 + 2$ This is the basic parabola moved up two units so that its vertex is at $(0,2)$. The points $(-1,3)$ and $(1,3)$ can be used to help sketch the parabola.

5. $y = 4x^2$ This parabola has its vertex at the origin and opens upward. It is narrower than the basic parabola. The points $(-1,4)$ and $(1,4)$ can be used to help sketch the parabola.

9. $y = \frac{1}{3}x^2$ This parabola has its vertex at the origin and opens upward. It is wider than the basic parabola. The points $(-2,\frac{4}{3})$ and $(2,\frac{4}{3})$ can be used to help sketch the parabola.

13. $y = (x-1)^2$ This is the basic parabola shifted one unit to the right so that its vertex is at $(1,0)$. The points $(0,1)$ and $(2,1)$ can be used to help sketch the parabola.

17. $y = 3x^2 + 2$ This parabola has its vertex at $(0,2)$ and opens upward. It is narrower than the basic parabola. The points $(-1,5)$ and $(1,5)$ can be used to help sketch the parabola. It can also be viewed as the parabola $y = 3x^2$ moved up two units.

21. $y = (x-1)^2 - 2$ This is the basic parabola shifted one unit to the right and two units down so that its vertex is at $(1,-2)$. The points $(0,-1)$ and $(2,-1)$ can be used to help sketch the parabola.

25. $y = 3(x-2)^2 - 4$ This parabola has its vertex at $(2,-4)$ and opens upward. It is narrower than the basic parabola. The points $(1,-1)$ and $(3,-1)$ can be used to help sketch the parabola.

29. $y = -\frac{1}{2}(x+1)^2 - 2$ This parabola has its vertex at $(-1,-2)$ and opens downward. It is wider than the basic parabola. The points $(-3,-4)$ and $(1,-4)$ can be used to help sketch the parabola.

Problem Set 7.7

1. $y = x^2 - 6x + 13 = x^2 - 6x + 9 + 13 - 9 = (x-3)^2 + 4$

This is the basic parabola shifted three units to the right and four units up so that its vertex is at $(3,4)$. The points $(2,5)$ and $(4,5)$ can be used to help sketch the parabola.

5. $y = x^2 - 5x + 3 = x^2 - 5x + \frac{25}{4} + 3 - \frac{25}{4} = (x - \frac{5}{2})^2 - \frac{13}{4}$

This is the basic parabola shifted $2\frac{1}{2}$ units to the right and $3\frac{1}{4}$ units down so that its vertex is at $(\frac{5}{2}, -\frac{13}{4})$. The points $(1,-1)$ and $(4,-1)$ can be used to help sketch the parabola.

9. $y = 3x^2 - 6x + 5$

$= 3(x^2 - 2x \quad) + 5$ Factor a 3 from the first two terms.

$= 3(x^2 - 2x + 1) + 5 - 3$ Add 1 inside the parentheses to complete the square. Subtract 3 to compensate for the 1 added inside the parentheses times the factor of 3.

$= 3(x-1)^2 + 2$

This parabola has its vertex at $(1,2)$ and opens upward. It is narrower than the basic parabola. The points $(0,5)$ and $(2,5)$ can be used to help sketch the parabola.

13. $y = -2x^2 - 4x - 5$

$= -2(x^2 + 2x \quad) - 5$ Factor -2 from the first two terms.

$= -2(x^2 + 2x + 1) - 5 + 2$ Add 1 inside the parentheses to complete the square.

$= -2(x+1)^2 - 3$ Add 2 to compensate for the 1 added inside the parentheses times a factor of -2.

This parabola has its vertex at $(-1,-3)$ and opens downward. It is narrower than the basic parabola. The points $(-2,-5)$ and $(0,-5)$ can be used to help sketch the parabola.

17. $y = 2x^2-x+2$

$$= 2(x^2 - \tfrac{1}{2}x \qquad) + 2$$

$$= 2(x^2 - \tfrac{1}{2}x + \tfrac{1}{16}) + 2 - \tfrac{1}{8}$$

$$= 2(x - \tfrac{1}{4})^2 + \tfrac{15}{8}$$

This basic parabola has its vertex at $(\tfrac{1}{4}, \tfrac{15}{8})$ and opens upward. It is narrower than the basic parabola. The points $(-1,5)$ and $(\tfrac{3}{2},5)$ can be used to help sketch the parabola.

21. $y = -3x^2-7x-2$

$$= -3(x^2 + \tfrac{7}{3}x + \tfrac{49}{36}) - 2 + \tfrac{49}{12}$$

$$= -3(x + \tfrac{7}{6})^2 + \tfrac{25}{12}$$

This parabola has its vertex at $(-\tfrac{7}{6}, \tfrac{25}{12})$ and opens downward. It is narrower than the basic parabola. The points $(-\tfrac{7}{3},-2)$ and $(0,-2)$ can be used to help sketch the parabola.

25. $\qquad x^2+y^2+6x+10y+18 = 0$

$$x^2+6x + \underline{\quad} + y^2+10y + \underline{\quad} = -18$$

$$x^2+6x+9+y^2+10y+25 = -18+9+25$$

$$(x+3)^2+(y+5)^2 = 4^2$$

The center is at $(-3,-5)$ and the length of a radius is 4 units.

29. $\qquad x^2+y^2-16x+6y+71 = 0$

$$x^2-16x + \underline{\quad} + y^2+6y + \underline{\quad} = -71$$

$$x^2-16x+64+y^2+6y+9 = -71+64+9$$

$$(x-8)^2+(y+3)^2 = (\sqrt{2})^2$$

The center is at $(8,-3)$ and the length of a radius is $\sqrt{2}$ units.

33. $\qquad 4x^2+4y^2+4x-32y+33 = 0$

$$4(x^2+x + \underline{\quad}) + 4(y^2-8y + \underline{\quad}) = -33$$

$$4(x^2+x + \tfrac{1}{4}) + 4(y^2-8y+16) = -33+1+64$$

$$4(x + \tfrac{1}{2})^2 + 4(y-4)^2 = 32$$

$$(x + \tfrac{1}{2})^2 + (y-4)^2 = 8$$

$$(x + \tfrac{1}{2})^2 + (y-4)^2 = (2\sqrt{2})^2$$

The center is at $(-\tfrac{1}{2},4)$ and the length of a radius is $2\sqrt{2}$ units.

37. Substitute -4 for h, 1 for k, and 8 for r in the form $(x-h)^2+(y-k)^2 = r^2$ and simplify.

$$(x-h)^2+(y-k)^2 = r^2$$
$$(x-(-4))^2+(y-1)^2 = 8^2$$
$$(x+4)^2+(y-1)^2 = 8^2$$
$$x^2+8x+16+y^2-2y+1 = 64$$
$$x^2+y^2+8x-2y-47 = 0$$

41. Substitute 0 for h, 0 for k, and $2\sqrt{5}$ for r.

$$(x-h)^2+(y-k)^2 = r^2$$
$$(x-0)^2+(y-0)^2 = (2\sqrt{5})^2$$
$$x^2+y^2 = 20$$
$$x^2+y^2-20 = 0$$

45. If the center is at (0,4) and the circle passes through the origin, then a radius must be 4 units long. Therefore, we can substitute 0 for h, 4 for k, and 4 for r.

$$(x-h)^2+(y-k)^2 = r^2$$
$$(x-0)^2+(y-4)^2 = 4^2$$
$$x^2+y^2-8y+16 = 16$$
$$x^2+y^2-8y = 0$$

Problem Set 7.8

The key idea for Problems 1-20, inclusive, is to be able to recognize the equations of ellipses and hyperbolas.

ellipse: The graph of $Ax^2+By^2 = C$ is an ellipse if A,B, and C are of the same sign and $A \neq B$.

hyperbola: The graph of $Ax^2+By^2 = C$ is a hyperbola if A,B, and C are nonzero constants and A and B are of unlike signs.

1. $x^2+4y^2 = 36$ Since A,B, and C are of like signs and $A \neq B$, this is an ellipse.

Let $x = 0$; then $0^2+4y^2 = 36$
$$4y^2 = 36$$
$$y^2 = 9$$
$$y = \pm 3.$$

The points (0,3) and (0,-3) are the endpoints of the minor axis.

Let $y = 0$; then $x^2+4(0)^2 = 36$
$$x^2 = 36$$
$$x = \pm 6.$$

The points (6,0) and (-6,0) are the endpoints of the major axis.

5. $x^2-y^2 = 1$ Since A and B are of unlike signs, it is a hyperbola.

Let $x = 0$; then $-y^2 = 1$
$$y^2 = -1.$$

Since $y^2 = -1$ has no real number solution, the hyperbola has no points on the y-axis.

Let $y = 0$; then $x^2 = 1$
$$x = \pm 1.$$

The points $(1,0)$ and $(-1,0)$ are on the graph.

The equations of the asymptotes can be found as follows.
$$x^2-y^2 = 0$$
$$-y^2 = -x^2$$
$$y^2 = x^2$$
$$y = \pm x$$

Thus, the lines $y = x$ and $y = -x$ are the asymptotes.

9. $4x^2+3y^2 = 12$ Since A,B, and C are of the same sign and $A \neq B$, this is an ellipse.

Let $x = 0$; then $3y^2 = 12$
$$y^2 = 4$$
$$y = \pm 2.$$

The points $(0,2)$ and $(0,-2)$ are the endpoints of the major axis.

Let $y = 0$; then $4x^2 = 12$
$$x^2 = 3$$
$$x = \pm \sqrt{3}.$$

The points $(\sqrt{3},0)$ and $(-\sqrt{3},0)$ are the endpoints of the minor axis.

13. $25x^2+2y^2 = 50$ Since A,B, and C are of the same sign and $A \neq B$, this is an ellipse.

Let $x = 0$; then $2y^2 = 50$
$$y^2 = 25$$
$$y = \pm 5.$$

The points $(0,5)$ and $(0,-5)$ are endpoints of the major axis.

Let $y = 0$; then $25x^2 = 50$
$$x^2 = 2$$
$$x = \pm \sqrt{2}.$$

The points $(-\sqrt{2},0)$ and $(\sqrt{2},0)$ are endpoints of the minor axis.

17. $-4x^2+y^2 = -4$ or $4x^2-y^2 = 4$ Since the signs of A and B are different, this is a hyperbola.

Let $x = 0$; then $-y^2 = 4$
$$y^2 = -4.$$

Since $y^2 = -4$ has no real solutions, there are no points of this hyperbola on the y-axis.

Let $y = 0$; then $4x^2 = 4$
$$x^2 = 1$$
$$x = \pm 1.$$

The points $(1,0)$ and $(-1,0)$ are on the graph.

The asymptotes can be found as follows.
$$4x^2-y^2 = 0$$
$$-y^2 = -4x^2$$
$$y^2 = 4x^2$$
$$y = \pm 2x$$

The equations of the asymptotes are $y = 2x$ and $y = -2x$.

21. Notice that x cannot equal zero and y cannot equal zero for each of these equations. Thus, there are no points on either axis. You will need to plot a sufficient number of points to determine these hyperbolas.

Chapter 8

Problem Set 8.1

1. The domain is the set of all first components of the ordered pairs.
    Domain = {1,2,3,4}

    The range is the set of all second components of the ordered pairs.
    Range = {5,8,11,14}

    It is a function because no two ordered pairs have the same first element.

5. Domain = {1,2,3,4,5}

    Range = {2,5,10,17,26}

    It is a function because no two ordered pairs have the same first element.

9. Domain = {all reals}

    Range = {nonnegative reals}

    Since $y = \sqrt[3]{x^2}$, to each member of the domain there will be assigned only one member of the range. Thus, it is a function.

13. $f(x) = \dfrac{1}{x-1}$ The denominator cannot equal zero; therefore, x cannot equal 1. So the domain is
    $$D = \{x \mid x \neq 1\}.$$

17. $h(x) = \dfrac{2}{(x+1)(x-4)}$ The denominator cannot equal zero; thus, x cannot equal -1 nor 4. The domain is
    $$D = \{x \mid x \neq -1 \text{ and } x \neq 4\}.$$

21. $f(x) = \dfrac{-4}{x^2+6x}$
    $$x^2+6x = 0$$
    $$x(x+6) = 0$$
    $$x = 0 \text{ or } x+6 = 0$$
    $$x = 0 \text{ or } \quad x = -6$$
    $$D = \{x \mid x \neq 0 \text{ and } x \neq -6\}.$$

25. $f(t) = \dfrac{3t}{t^2-4}$
    $$t^2-4 = 0$$
    $$t^2 = 4$$
    $$t = \pm 2$$
    $$D = \{t \mid t \neq -2 \text{ and } t \neq 2\}.$$

29. $f(s) = \sqrt{4s-5}$
    $$4s-5 \geq 0$$
    $$4s \geq 5$$
    $$s \geq \frac{5}{4}$$
    $$D = \{s \mid s \geq \tfrac{5}{4}\}.$$

33. $f(x) = \sqrt{x^2-3x-18} = \sqrt{(x-6)(x+3)}$

$(x-6)(x+3) \geq 0$

$(x-6)(x+3) = 0$ $(x-6)(x+3) = 0$

(-4)   (0)   (7)

-3		6
x-6 is negative. x+3 is negative. Their product is <u>positive</u>.	x-6 is negative. x+3 is positive. Their product is <u>negative</u>.	x-6 is positive. x+3 is positive. Their product is <u>positive</u>.

$D = \{x \mid x \leq -3 \text{ or } x \geq 6\}.$

37. $\underline{f(x) = 5x-2}$

$f(0) = 5(0)-2 = -2, \quad f(2) = 5(2)-2 = 8,$

$f(-1) = 5(-1)-2 = -7, \quad f(-4) = 5(-4)-2 = -22$

41. $\underline{g(x) = 2x^2-5x-7}$

$g(-1) = 2(-1)^2-5(-1)-7 = 2(1)+5-7 = 0$

$g(2) = 2(2)^2-5(2)-7 = 8-10-7 = -9$

$g(-3) = 2(-3)^2-5(-3)-7 = 18+15-7 = 26$

$g(4) = 2(4)^2-5(4)-7 = 32-20-7 = 5$

45. $\underline{f(x) = \sqrt{2x+1}}$

$f(3) = \sqrt{2(3)+1} = \sqrt{7}$

$f(4) = \sqrt{2(4)+1} = \sqrt{9} = 3$

$f(10) = \sqrt{2(10)+1} = \sqrt{21}$

$f(12) = \sqrt{2(12)+1} = \sqrt{25} = 5$

49. $\underline{f(x) = 5x^2-2x+3} \qquad \underline{g(x) = -x^2+4x-5}$

$f(-2) = 5(-2)^2-2(-2)+3 = 20+4+3 = 27$

$f(3) = 5(3)^2-2(3)+3 = 45-6+3 = 42$

$g(-4) = -(-4)^2+4(-4)-5 = -16-16-5 = -37$

$g(6) = -(6)^2+4(6)-5 = -36+24-5 = -17$

53. $\underline{f(x) = -3x+6}$

$f(a+h) = -3(a+h)+6 = -3a-3h+6$

$f(a) = -3(a)+6 = -3a+6$

$\dfrac{f(a+h)-f(a)}{h} = \dfrac{(-3a-3h+6)-(-3a+6)}{h}$

$= \dfrac{-3a-3h+6+3a-6}{h}$

$= \dfrac{-3h}{h} = -3$

57. $f(x) = 2x^2 - x + 8$

$f(a+h) = 2(a+h)^2 - (a+h) + 8 = 2a^2 + 4ah + h^2 - a - h + 8$

$f(a) = 2a^2 - a + 8$

$$\frac{f(a+h) - f(a)}{h} = \frac{(2a^2 + 4ah + 2h^2 - a - h + 8) - (2a^2 - a + 8)}{h}$$

$$= \frac{2a^2 + 4ah + 2h^2 - a - h + 8 - 2a^2 + a - 8}{h}$$

$$= \frac{4ah + 2h^2 - h}{h} = \frac{\cancel{h}(4a + 2h - 1)}{\cancel{h}} = 4a - 1 + 2h$$

61. $h(t) = 64t - 16t^2$ 65. $I(r) = 500r$

$h(1) = 64(1) - 16(1)^2 = 64 - 16 = 48$ $I(.11) = 55$

$h(2) = 64(2) - 16(2)^2 = 128 - 64 = 64$ $I(.12) = 60$

$h(3) = 64(3) - 16(3)^2 = 192 - 144 = 48$ $I(.135) = 67.5$

$h(4) = 64(4) - 16(4)^2 = 256 - 256 = 0$ $I(.15) = 75$

Problem Set 8.2

1.   We should recognize that $f(x) = 2x - 4$ is a linear function and thus its graph is a straight line. Two points are necessary to determine a straight line, but it is advisable to find a third point for checking purposes.

   $f(0) = 2(0) - 4 = -4$, $f(2) = 2(2) - 4 = 0$, $f(3) = 2(3) - 4 = 2$

   Plot the three points $(0,-4)$, $(2,0)$, and $(3,2)$ and draw the line determined by them.

5.   The function $f(x) = -3x$ is a linear function.

   $f(0) = 0$, $f(1) = -3$, $f(-2) = 6$

   Plot the points $(0,0)$, $(1,-3)$, and $(-2,6)$ and draw the line.

9.   The function $f(x) = -x + 3$ is a linear function.

   $f(0) = 3$, $f(3) = 0$, $f(1) = 2$

   Plot the points $(0,3)$, $(3,0)$, and $(1,2)$ and draw the line.

13.   The function $f(x) = -x^2 + 6x - 8$ is a quadratic function and thus its graph is a parabola. Remember that we have two basic approaches to graphing parabolas. Let's complete the square for this one.

$$f(x) = -x^2 + 6x - 8$$
$$= -(x^2 - 6x + \underline{}) - 8$$
$$= -(x^2 - 6x + 9) - 8 + 9$$
$$= -(x-3)^2 + 1$$

This parabola has its vertex at $(3,1)$ and opens downward. The points $(2,0)$ and $(4,0)$ can be used to help sketch the parabola.

17. The function $f(x) = 2x^2-20x+52$ is a quadratic function. Let's use the same approach as demonstrated in Examples 4 and 5 in the text.

Step 1: Since the coefficient of x^2 is positive, the parabola opens upward.

Step 2: $-\dfrac{b}{2a} = -\dfrac{-20}{4} = 5$

Step 3: $f(5) = 2(5)^2-20(5)+52 = 2$
Therefore, the vertex is at (5,2).

Step 4: Let $x = 4$; then $f(4) = 2(16)-20(4)+52 = 4$.
Thus, the point (4,4) and its reflection (6,4) across the line of symmetry $x = 5$ are both on the graph.

21. The function $f(x) = x^2-x+2$ is a quadratic function. Let's complete the square to help graph this one.

$$f(x) = x^2-x+2$$
$$= x^2 - x + \frac{1}{4} + 2 - \frac{1}{4}$$
$$= \left(x - \frac{1}{2}\right)^2 + \frac{7}{4}$$

The vertex is at $\left(\frac{1}{2}, \frac{7}{4}\right)$ and the parabola opens upward. The points (-1,4) and (2,4) can be used to help sketch the parabola.

25. The function $f(x) = -2x^2-1$ is a quadratic function. The vertex of the parabola is at (0,-1) and it opens downward. It is narrower than the basic parabola. The points (1,-3) and (-1,-3) can be used to help sketch the parabola.

29. The function $f(x) = -2x^2+14x-25$ is a quadratic function. Let's complete the square to help with this graph.

$$f(x) = -2x^2+14x-25$$
$$= -2(x^2-7x + \underline{}) -25$$
$$= -2\left(x^2-7x + \frac{49}{4}\right) - 25 + \frac{49}{2}$$
$$= -2\left(x - \frac{7}{2}\right)^2 - \frac{1}{2}$$

The vertex is at $\left(\frac{7}{2}, -\frac{1}{2}\right)$ and the parabola opens downward. It is narrower than the basic parabola. The points (2,-5) and (5,-5) can be used to help sketch the parabola.

33. $f(x) = \sqrt{x+2}$ This is the basic square root curve shifted to the left two units.

37. $f(x) = \sqrt{x+3} + 1$ This is the basic square root curve shifted three units to the left and one unit up.

41. $f(x) = |x|-1$ This is the basic absolute value graph shifted down one unit.

45. $f(x) = -|x-2|$ This is the basic absolute value graph reflected across the x-axis and shifted to the right two units.

49. $f(x) = 2|x|$ This is the basic absolute value graph except narrower. The points $(1,2)$ and $(-1,2)$ can be used to help with the sketch.

53. $f(x) = x^3$ Since this is a "new" curve, you will need to plot a sufficient number of points to determine it.

57. $f(x) = (x-3)^3$ This is the basic cubic curve shifted to the right three units.

61. $f(x) = -(x+3)^3+1$ This is the basic cubic curve reflected across the x-axis, shifted to the left three units, and shifted up one unit.

65. $f(x) = \dfrac{1}{x+1}$ This is the basic graph of $f(x) = \dfrac{1}{x}$ (Problem 62) shifted to the left one unit.

Problem Set 8.3

1. $C(x) = 2x^2-320x+12920$ The x-value of the vertex is given by $-\dfrac{b}{2a}$.

$$-\frac{b}{2a} = -\frac{-320}{4} = 80$$

80 items should be produced.

5.

$$\frac{240-2x}{2} = 120-x$$

The function $A(x) = x(120-x)$ represents the area of the rectangle in terms of the length x.

$$A = x(120-x) = -x^2+120x$$
$$-\frac{b}{2a} = -\frac{120}{-2} = 60$$

The length should be 60 meters and the width $120-60 = 60$ meters.

9. To evaluate $(f \circ g)(-2)$ we substitute -2 into the g function and this result is then substituted into the f function.

$(f \circ g)(-2) = f(-4(-2)+6) = f(14) = 9(14)-2 = 124$

To evaluate $(g \circ f)(4)$ we substitute 4 into the f function and this result is then substituted into the g function.

$(g \circ f)(4) = g(9(4)-2) = g(34) = -4(34)+6 = -130$

13. $(f \circ g)(2) = f(\frac{2}{2-1}) = f(2) = \frac{1}{2}$

$(g \circ f)(-1) = g(\frac{1}{-1}) = g(-1) = \frac{2}{-1-1} = \frac{2}{-2} = -1$

17. $(f \circ g)(1) = f(-1+4) = f(3) = \sqrt{3(3)-2} = \sqrt{7}$

$(g \circ f)(6) = g(\sqrt{3(6)-2}) = g(\sqrt{16}) = g(4) = -4+4 = 0$

21. $f(x) = 3x$ $g(x) = 5x-1$

$f(g(x)) = f(5x-1) = 3(5x-1) = 15x-3$

$g(f(x)) = g(3x) = 5(3x)-1 = 15x-1$

Since f and g are defined for all reals, so are f∘g and g∘f.

25. $f(x) = 3x+2$ $g(x) = x^2+3$

$f(g(x)) = f(x^2+3) = 3(x^2+3)+2 = 3x^2+11$

$g(f(x)) = g(3x+2) = (3x+2)^2+3 = 9x^2+12x+7$

Since f and g are defined for all reals, so are f∘g and g∘f.

29. $f(x) = \dfrac{3}{x}$ $g(x) = 4x-9$

$f(g(x)) = f(4x-9) = \dfrac{3}{4x-9}$

The domain of g is the set of all reals but the domain of f excludes 0.
Therefore, $4x-9 \neq 0$ or $x \neq \dfrac{9}{4}$. Thus, the domain of f∘g is $\{x \mid x \neq \dfrac{9}{4}\}$.

$g(f(x)) = g(\dfrac{3}{x}) = 4(\dfrac{3}{x})-9 = \dfrac{12}{x} - 9 = \dfrac{12-9x}{x}$

The domain of f excludes 0. Thus, the domain of g∘f is $\{x \mid x \neq 0\}$.

33. $f(x) = \dfrac{1}{x}$ $g(x) = \dfrac{1}{x-4}$ $f(g(x)) = f(\dfrac{1}{x-4}) = \dfrac{1}{\dfrac{1}{x-4}} = x-4$

The domain of g excludes 4. The domain of f excludes 0 so g(x), which is
$\dfrac{1}{x-4}$, cannot equal 0. The expression $\dfrac{1}{x-4}$ will never equal zero so the
initial restriction, $x \neq 4$, on the domain of g is sufficient. Thus, the
domain of f∘g is $\{x \mid x \neq 4\}$.

$$g(f(x)) = g(\dfrac{1}{x}) = \dfrac{1}{\dfrac{1}{x} - 4} = \dfrac{1}{\dfrac{1-4x}{x}} = \dfrac{x}{1-4x}$$

The domain of f excludes 0. Furthermore, since the domain of g excludes 4,
$f(x)$ (which is $\dfrac{1}{x}$) cannot equal 4. Thus, x cannot equal $\dfrac{1}{4}$. Therefore,
the domain of g∘f is $\{x \mid x \neq 0 \text{ and } x \neq \dfrac{1}{4}\}$.

37. $f(x) = \dfrac{3}{2x}$ $g(x) = \dfrac{1}{x+1}$

$$f(g(x)) = f(\dfrac{1}{x+1}) = \dfrac{3}{2(\dfrac{1}{x+1})} = \dfrac{3}{\dfrac{2}{x+1}} = \dfrac{3(x+1)}{2} = \dfrac{3x+3}{2}$$

The domain of g excludes -1. The domain of f excludes 0 so g(x), which is
$\dfrac{1}{x+1}$, cannot equal 0. The expression $\dfrac{1}{x+1}$ will never equal zero, so the
initial restriction, $x \neq -1$, on the domain of g is sufficient. Thus, the
domain of f∘g is $\{x \mid x \neq -1\}$.

$$g(f(x)) = g(\frac{3}{2x}) = \frac{1}{\frac{3}{2x}+1} = \frac{1}{\frac{3+2x}{2x}} = \frac{2x}{3+2x}$$

The domain of f excludes 0. Since the domain of g excludes -1, f(x) (which is $\frac{3}{2x}$) cannot equal -1. Thus, x cannot equal $-\frac{3}{2}$. Therefore, the domain of g∘f is $\{x \mid x \neq 0 \text{ and } x \neq -\frac{3}{2}\}$.

41. $f(x) = 4x+2$ $g(x) = \frac{x-2}{4}$

$$f(g(x)) = f(\frac{x-2}{4}) = 4(\frac{x-2}{4})+2 = x-2+2 = x$$

$$g(f(x)) = g(4x+2) = \frac{4x+2-2}{4} = \frac{4x}{4} = x$$

45. $f(x) = -\frac{1}{4}x - \frac{1}{2}$ $g(x) = -4x-2$

$$f(g(x)) = f(-4x-2) = -\frac{1}{4}(-4x-2) - \frac{1}{2}$$
$$= x + \frac{1}{2} - \frac{1}{2} = x$$

$$g(f(x)) = g(-\frac{1}{4}x - \frac{1}{2}) = -4(-\frac{1}{4}x - \frac{1}{2}) - 2$$
$$= x+2-2$$
$$= x$$

Problem Set 8.4

1. Some vertical lines will intersect the graph in more than one point; thus, the graph does not exhibit a function.

5. No vertical line will intersect the graph in more than one point. Thus, the graph exhibits a function.

9. No horizontal line will intersect the graph in more than one point. Thus, the graph exhibits a one-to-one function.

13. Some horizontal lines will intersect the graph in more than one point. Thus, the graph does not exhibit a one-to-one function.

17. The domain of f consists of the set of first components of the given ordered pairs. The range of f is the set of second components of the ordered pairs. The inverse of f can be formed by switching the components of all of the ordered pairs of f.

21. $f(x) = 5x-4$ The f function "multiplies a number by 5 and then subtracts 4." The inverse function should "add 4 and then divide by 5." Therefore,
$$f^{-1}(x) = \frac{x+4}{5} \ .$$

$$f(f^{-1}(x)) = f(\frac{x+4}{5}) = 5(\frac{x+4}{5})-4 = x+4-4 = x$$

$$f^{-1}(x)) = f^{-1}(5x-4) = \frac{5x-4+4}{5} = \frac{5x}{5} = x$$

25. $f(x) = \frac{4}{5}x$ The f function "multiplies a number by $\frac{4}{5}$." The inverse function should "divide by $\frac{4}{5}$" which is equivalent to multiplying by $\frac{5}{4}$. Therefore,
$$f^{-1}(x) = \frac{5}{4}x.$$

$$f(f^{-1}(x)) = f\left(\tfrac{5}{4}x\right) = \tfrac{4}{5}\left(\tfrac{5}{4}x\right) = x$$

$$f^{-1}(f(x)) = f^{-1}\left(\tfrac{4}{5}x\right) = \tfrac{5}{4}\left(\tfrac{4}{5}x\right) = x$$

29. $f(x) = \dfrac{1}{3}x - \dfrac{2}{5}$ The f function "multiplies a number by $\tfrac{1}{3}$ and then subtracts $\tfrac{2}{5}$." The inverse function should "add $\tfrac{2}{5}$ and then divide by $\tfrac{1}{3}$."
Therefore,

$$f^{-1}(x) = \dfrac{x + \tfrac{2}{5}}{\tfrac{1}{3}} = 3\left(x + \tfrac{2}{5}\right) = 3x + \tfrac{6}{5} = \dfrac{15x+6}{5}$$

$$f(f^{-1}(x)) = f\left(\dfrac{15x+6}{5}\right) = \tfrac{1}{3}\left(\dfrac{15x+6}{5}\right) - \tfrac{2}{5} = \dfrac{15x+6}{15} - \dfrac{6}{15} = \dfrac{15x}{15} = x$$

$$f^{-1}(f(x)) = f^{-1}\left(\tfrac{1}{3}x - \tfrac{2}{5}\right) = \dfrac{15\left(\tfrac{1}{3}x - \tfrac{2}{5}\right) + 6}{5}$$

$$= \dfrac{5x-6+6}{5} = \dfrac{5x}{5} = x$$

33. $f(x) = -5x - 4$

Substitute y for f(x), exchange variables, and solve for y.

$$y = -5x-4$$
$$x = -5y-4$$
$$5y = -4-x$$
$$y = \dfrac{-4-x}{5}$$

Therefore, $f^{-1}(x) = \dfrac{-4-x}{5}$.

$$f(f^{-1}(x)) = f\left(\dfrac{-4-x}{5}\right) = -5\left(\dfrac{-4-x}{5}\right) - 4$$
$$= 4+x-4 = x$$

$$f^{-1}(f(x)) = f^{-1}(-5x-4) = \dfrac{-4-(-5x-4)}{5} = \dfrac{-4+5x+4}{5} = \dfrac{5x}{5} = x$$

37. $f(x) = \dfrac{4}{3}x - \dfrac{1}{4}$

Substitute y for f(x), exchange variables, and solve for y.

$$y = \dfrac{4}{3}x - \dfrac{1}{4}$$
$$x = \dfrac{4}{3}y - \dfrac{1}{4}$$
$$12x = 16y-3$$
$$12x+3 = 16y$$
$$\dfrac{12x+3}{16} = y$$
$$\dfrac{3}{4}x + \dfrac{3}{16} = y$$

Therefore, $f^{-1}(x) = \dfrac{3}{4}x + \dfrac{3}{16}$.

$$f(f^{-1}(x)) = f(\tfrac{3}{4}x + \tfrac{3}{16}) = \tfrac{4}{3}(\tfrac{3}{4}x + \tfrac{3}{16}) - \tfrac{1}{4}$$

$$= x + \tfrac{1}{4} - \tfrac{1}{4} = x$$

$$f^{-1}(f(x)) = f^{-1}(\tfrac{4}{3}x - \tfrac{1}{4}) = \tfrac{3}{4}(\tfrac{4}{3}x - \tfrac{1}{4}) + \tfrac{3}{16}$$

$$= x - \tfrac{3}{16} + \tfrac{3}{16} = x$$

41. $f(x) = 4x$

Substitute y for f(x), exchange variables, and solve for y.

$$y = 4x$$
$$x = 4y$$
$$\frac{x}{4} = y$$

Therefore, $f^{-1}(x) = \tfrac{1}{4}x.$

45. $f(x) = 3x-3$

Substitute y for f(x), exchange variables, and solve for y.

$$y = 3x-3$$
$$x = 3y-3$$
$$x+3 = 3y$$
$$\frac{x+3}{3} = y$$

Therefore, $f^{-1}(x) = \frac{x+3}{3}.$

49. $f(x) = x^2,\ x \geq 0$

Substitute y for f(x), exchange variables, and solve for y.

$$y = x^2$$
$$x = y^2$$
$$\sqrt{x} = y$$

Therefore, $f^{-1}(x) = \sqrt{x},\ x \geq 0.$

<u>Problem Set 8.5</u>

13. $y = kx^2$ represents the direct variation.

Now we can substitute −144 for y, 6 for x, and solve for k.

$$-144 = 36k$$
$$-\frac{144}{36} = k$$
$$-4 = k$$

17. $y = \dfrac{k}{x}$ represents the inverse variation.

Now we can substitute -4 for y, $\dfrac{1}{2}$ for x, and solve for k.

$$-4 = \dfrac{k}{\dfrac{1}{2}}$$

$$k = -2$$

21. $y = \dfrac{kx}{z}$ represents the direct and inverse variation. Now we can substitute 2 for z, 45 for y, 18 for x, and solve for k.

$$45 = \dfrac{18k}{2}$$
$$45 = 9k$$
$$5 = k$$

25. $y = kx$ represents the direct variation.

We can substitute 36 for y, 48 for x, and solve for k.

$$36 = 48k$$
$$\dfrac{36}{48} = k$$
$$\dfrac{3}{4} = k$$

Therefore, the specific equation is $y = \dfrac{3}{4}x$. Now we can substitute 12 for x to determine y.

$$y = \dfrac{3}{4}(12) = 9$$

29. $A = kbh$ represents the joint variation. We can substitute 60 for A, 12 for b, 10 for h, and solve for k.

$$60 = k(12)(10)$$
$$60 = 120k$$
$$\dfrac{60}{120} = k$$
$$\dfrac{1}{2} = k$$

The specific equation is $A = \dfrac{1}{2}bh$. Now we can substitute 16 for b and 14 for h to determine A.

$$A = \dfrac{1}{2}(16)(14) = 112$$

33. $V = \dfrac{kT}{P}$ represents the direct and inverse variation. We can substitute 48 for V, 320 for T, 20 for P, and solve for k.

$$48 = \dfrac{k(320)}{20}$$
$$48 = 16k$$
$$3 = k$$

The specific equation is $V = \dfrac{3T}{P}$. Now we can substitute 280 for T and 30 for P to determine V.

$$V = \dfrac{3(280)}{30} = 28$$

37. $R = \dfrac{k\ell}{d^2}$ represents the direct and inverse variations. We can substitute 1.5 for R, .5 for d, 20000 for ℓ (200 meters = 20000 centimeters), and solve for k.

$$1.5 = \frac{20000k}{.25}$$

$$1.5 = 80000k$$

$$\frac{1.5}{80000} = k$$

$$\frac{3}{160000} = k$$

The specific equation is $R = \dfrac{\dfrac{3}{160000}\,\ell}{d^2}$ or $R = \dfrac{3\ell}{160000d^2}$. Now we can substitute 40000 for ℓ and .25 for d to determine R.

$$R = \frac{3(40000)}{160000(.25)^2}$$

$$R = 12$$

Chapter 9

Problem Set 9.1

1. Graph the two lines on the same set of axes. The coordinates of the point of intersection of the two lines should be (3,2). You should check these coordinates in both equations.

5. The two equations should produce the same line. Thus, the equations are said to be dependent. Any solution of one equation is also a solution of the other equation.

9. The graphs of the two equations should be parallel lines. Thus, there is no point of intersection, which means no solution for the system. The solution set is $\emptyset$.

13. $4x+3y = -40$ Leave alone. $4x+3y = -40$

$5x - y = -12$ Multiply by 3. $15x-3y = -36$

$$19x \quad = -76$$
$$x = -4$$

Substitute -4 for x in either of the two original equations.

$$5x-y = -12$$
$$5(-4)-y = -12$$
$$-y = 8$$
$$y = -8$$

The solution set is $\{(-4,-8)\}$.

17. $4x - 5y = 3$ Multiply by 3. $12x-15y = 9$

$8x+15y = -24$ Leave alone. $8x+15y = -24$

$$20x \quad = -15$$
$$x = -\frac{15}{20}$$
$$x = -\frac{3}{4}$$

Substitute $-\frac{3}{4}$ for x in either of the two original equations.

$$4x-5y = 3$$
$$4\left(-\frac{3}{4}\right)-5y = 3$$
$$-3-5y = 3$$
$$-5y = 6$$
$$y = -\frac{6}{5}$$

The solution set is $\left\{\left(-\frac{3}{4}, -\frac{6}{5}\right)\right\}$.

21. $9x+4y = 48$ Multiply by 7. $63x+28y = 336$

$5x-7y = 82$ Multiply by 4. $20x-28y = 328$

$$83x \quad = 664$$
$$x = 8$$

Substitute 8 for x in either of the two original equations.

$$9x+4y = 48$$
$$9(8)+4y = 48$$
$$4y = -24$$
$$y = -6$$

The solution set is $\{(8,-6)\}$.

25. $\quad \frac{1}{2}x - \frac{1}{3}y = 12 \quad$ <u>Multiply by 2.</u> $\longrightarrow \quad x - \frac{2}{3}y = 24$

$\quad \frac{3}{4}x + \frac{2}{3}y = 4 \quad$ <u>Leave alone.</u> $\longrightarrow \quad \dfrac{\frac{3}{4}x + \frac{2}{3}y = 4}{1\frac{3}{4}x \qquad = 28}$

$$\frac{7}{4}x = 28$$
$$x = 16$$

Substitute 16 for x in either of the two original equations.

$$\frac{1}{2}x - \frac{1}{3}y = 12$$
$$\frac{1}{2}(16) - \frac{1}{3}y = 12$$
$$-\frac{1}{3}y = 4$$
$$y = -12$$

The solution set is $\{(16,-12)\}$.

29. $\quad \dfrac{4x}{5} - \dfrac{3y}{2} = \dfrac{1}{5} \quad$ Multiply by $\frac{2}{3}$. $\longrightarrow \quad \dfrac{8x}{15} - y = \dfrac{2}{15}$

$\quad -2x + y = -1 \quad$ <u>Leave alone.</u> $\longrightarrow \quad \dfrac{-2x + y = -1}{-\dfrac{22x}{15} = -\dfrac{13}{15}}$

$$x = \frac{13}{22}$$

Substitute $\frac{13}{22}$ for x in either of the two original equations.

$$-2x+y = -1$$
$$-2\left(\frac{13}{22}\right)+y = -1$$
$$y = \frac{2}{11}$$

The solution set is $\{(\frac{13}{22},\frac{2}{11})\}$.

33. Let x represent the amount invested at 8% and y the amount invested at 9%.

$$x + y = 1000 \longrightarrow \text{total amount invested was } \$1000$$
$$.08x+.09y = 87 \longrightarrow \text{total income was } \$87.$$

Solving this system produces x = 300 and y = 700. Thus, $300 was invested at 8% and $700 at 9%.

37. Let g represent the cost of 1 golf ball and t the cost of one tennis ball.

The cost of 3 tennis balls and 2 golf balls is $7. $\longrightarrow$ $3t+2g = 7$

The cost of 6 tennis balls and 3 golf balls is $12. $\longrightarrow$ $6t+3g = 12$

Solving this system produces $t = 1$ and $g = 2$. Thus, the cost of one tennis ball is $1 and the cost of one golf ball is $2.

41. Let s represent the price of a student ticket and n the price of a non-student ticket.

3000 tickets were sold. $\longrightarrow$ $s+n = 3000$

The total income was $10000. $\longrightarrow$ $3s+5n = 10000$

Solving this system produces $s = 2500$ and $n = 500$. Thus, 2500 student tickets and 500 nonstudent tickets were sold.

Problem Set 9.2

1. $\begin{pmatrix} x+y = 20 \\ x = y-4 \end{pmatrix}$

The second equation indicates that y-4 can be substituted for x in the first equation.

$x+y = 20$ <u>Substitute y-4 for x.</u> $\longrightarrow$ $(y-4)+y = 20$

Solving this equation for y yields

$$y-4+y = 20$$
$$2y = 24$$
$$y = 12.$$

Now we can substitute 12 for y in $x = y-4$.

$$x = y-4$$
$$= 12-4$$
$$= 8$$

The solution set is $\{(8,12)\}$.

5. $\begin{pmatrix} x = -3y \\ 7x-2y = -69 \end{pmatrix}$

The first equation indicates that -3y can be substituted for x in the second equation.

$7x-2y = -69$ <u>Substitute -3y for x.</u> $\longrightarrow$ $7(-3y)-2y = -69$

We can solve this equation for y.

$$7(-3y)-2y = -69$$
$$-21y-2y = -69$$
$$-23y = -69$$
$$y = 3$$

Now we can substitute 3 for y in $x = -3y$.

$$x = -3y$$
$$x = -3(3) = -9$$

The solution set is $\{(-9,3)\}$.

9. $\begin{pmatrix} 2x+3y &= 11 \\ 3x-2y &= -3 \end{pmatrix}$

Let's solve the first equation for y in terms of x.

$$2x+3y = 11$$
$$3y = 11-2x$$
$$y = \frac{11-2x}{3}$$

Now we can substitute $\frac{11-2x}{3}$ for y in the second equation and solve for x.

$$3x-2y = -3$$
$$3x-2\left(\frac{11-2x}{3}\right) = -3$$
$$3x-\left(\frac{22-4x}{3}\right) = -3$$
$$9x-22+4x = -9$$
$$13x = 13$$
$$x = 1$$

Finally, let's substitute 1 for x in $y = \frac{11-2x}{3}$.

$$y = \frac{11-2(1)}{3} = \frac{11-2}{3} = \frac{9}{3} = 3$$

The solution set is $\{(1,3)\}$.

13. $\begin{pmatrix} y = \frac{2}{5}x-1 \\ 3x+5y = 4 \end{pmatrix}$

The first equation indicates that $\frac{2}{5}x-1$ can be substituted for y in the second equation.

$$3x+5y = 4$$
$$3x+5\left(\frac{2}{5}x-1\right) = 4$$
$$3x+2x-5 = 4$$
$$5x = 9$$
$$x = \frac{9}{5}$$

Now we can substitute $\frac{9}{5}$ for x in $y = \frac{2}{5}x-1$.

$$y = \frac{2}{5}\left(\frac{9}{5}\right)-1 = \frac{18}{25}-1 = -\frac{7}{25}$$

The solution set is $\{(\frac{9}{5}, -\frac{7}{25})\}$.

17. $\begin{pmatrix} 5x+3y = -7 \\ 7x-3y = 55 \end{pmatrix}$ Since the coefficients of the y-terms are opposites, let's add the two equations.

$$5x+3y = -7$$
$$\underline{7x-3y = 55}$$
$$12x \quad = 48$$
$$x = 4$$

Now we can substitute 4 for x in either of the two original equations.

$$5x+3y = -7$$
$$5(4)+3y = -7$$
$$3y = -27$$
$$y = 9$$

The solution set is $\{(4,-9)\}$.

21. $\begin{pmatrix} x = -6y+79 \\ x = 4y-41 \end{pmatrix}$

We can equate the two expressions for x from the equations.

$$-6y+79 = 4y-41$$
$$120 = 10y$$
$$12 = y$$

Now we can substitute 12 for y in either of the two original equations.

$$x = -6y+79$$
$$= -6(12)+79 = 7$$

The solution set is $\{(7,12)\}$.

25. $\begin{array}{l} 5x-2y = 1 \\ 10x-4y = 7 \end{array}$ $\quad \underrightarrow{\text{Multiply by } -2.}$ $\quad \underrightarrow{\text{Leave alone.}}$ $\quad \begin{array}{l} -10x+4y = -2 \\ \underline{10x-4y = 7} \\ 0 = 5 \end{array}$

The false statement $0 = 5$ implies that the system is inconsistent; its solution set is $\emptyset$.

29. $\begin{pmatrix} -2x+5y = -16 \\ x = \dfrac{3}{4}y+1 \end{pmatrix}$

The second equation indicates that $\dfrac{3}{4}y+1$ can be substituted for x in the first equation.

$$-2\left(\frac{3}{4}y+1\right)+5y = -16$$
$$-\frac{3}{2}y-2+5y = -16$$
$$-3y-4+10y = -32$$
$$7y = -28$$
$$y = -4$$

Now we can substitute -4 for y in $x = \dfrac{3}{4}y+1$.

$$x = \frac{3}{4}(-4)+1 = -2$$

The solution set is $\{(-2,-4)\}$.

33. $\dfrac{x}{6} + \dfrac{y}{3} = 3$ $\quad \underrightarrow{\text{Leave alone.}}$ $\quad \dfrac{x}{6} + \dfrac{y}{3} = 3$

$\dfrac{5x}{2} - \dfrac{y}{6} = -17$ $\quad \underrightarrow{\text{Multiply by } 2.}$ $\quad 5x - \dfrac{y}{3} = -34$

$$\frac{x}{6} + 5x = -31$$
$$\frac{31}{6}x = -31$$
$$x = -6$$

Now we can substitute -6 for x in either of the two original equations.

$$\frac{x}{6} + \frac{y}{3} = 3$$
$$\frac{-6}{6} + \frac{y}{3} = 3$$
$$-1 + \frac{y}{3} = 3$$
$$\frac{y}{3} = 4$$
$$y = 12$$

The solution set is $\{(-6,12)\}$.

37. $\begin{pmatrix} 5(x+1)-(y+3) = -6 \\ 2(x-2)+3(y-1) = 0 \end{pmatrix}$

First, let's simplify each of the equations.

$\begin{pmatrix} 5x+5-y-3 = -6 \\ 2x-4+3y-3 = 0 \end{pmatrix}$

$\begin{pmatrix} 5x - y = -8 \\ 2x+3y = 7 \end{pmatrix}$

Now let's use the elimination by addition method.

$$5x - y = -8 \quad \underline{\text{Multiply by 3.}} \longrightarrow \quad 15x-3y = -24$$
$$2x+3y = 7 \quad \underline{\text{Leave alone.}} \longrightarrow \quad \underline{2x+3y = \ \ 7}$$
$$17x \quad\ \ = -17$$
$$x = -1$$

Now we can substitute -1 for x in 5x-y = -8.

$$5(-1)-y = -8$$
$$-y = -3$$
$$y = 3$$

The solution set is $\{(-1,3)\}$.

Don't forget that to check this answer you need to substitute back into the original system.

41. $\begin{pmatrix} \dfrac{3x+y}{2} + \dfrac{x-2y}{5} = 8 \\ \dfrac{x-y}{3} - \dfrac{x+y}{6} = \dfrac{10}{3} \end{pmatrix}$

Multiply the first equation by 10 and the second equation by 6.

$\begin{pmatrix} 5(3x+y)+2(x-2y) = 80 \\ 2(x-y) - (x+y) = 20 \end{pmatrix}$

Simplify both equations.

$\begin{pmatrix} 15x+5y+2x-4y = 80 \\ 2x-2y - x - y = 20 \end{pmatrix}$

$\begin{pmatrix} 17x + y = 80 \\ x - 3y = 20 \end{pmatrix}$

Now we can solve this equivalent system by the elimination method.

$$17x+y = 80 \quad \underline{\text{Multiply by 3.}} \longrightarrow \quad 51x+3y = 240$$
$$x-3y = 20 \quad \underline{\text{Leave alone.}} \longrightarrow \quad \underline{x-3y = \ \ 20}$$
$$52x \quad\ \ = 260$$
$$x = 5$$

Now we can substitute 5 for x in 17+y = 80.

$$17(5)+y = 80$$
$$y = -5$$

The solution set is $\{(5,-5)\}$.

45. Let t represent the tens digit and u the units digit.

The sum of the digits is 11. $\longrightarrow$ t+u = 11

The tens digit is 1 more than
four times the units digit. $\longrightarrow$ t = 4u+1

Solving the system $\begin{pmatrix} t+u = 11 \\ t = 4u+1 \end{pmatrix}$ produces t = 9 and u = 2. Therefore, the number is 92.

49. Let x be the amount invested at 13% and y the amount at 15%.

A total of $600 was invested. $\longrightarrow$ x+y = 600

The income from the 15%
investment was $8 more
than twice the income
from the 13% investment. $\longrightarrow$ .15y = 2(.13x)+8

Solving the system $\begin{pmatrix} x+y = 600 \\ -.26x + .15y = 8 \end{pmatrix}$ produces x = 200 and y = 400.

53. Let t represent the tens digit and u the units digit. Then the original number is represented by 10t+u and the number with the digits reversed is represented by 10u+t.

The number divided by the sum of its digits is 2. $\longrightarrow$ $\dfrac{10t+u}{t+u} = 2$

This equation simplifies to 8t−u = 0.

The number formed by reversing the digits is 9
less than five times the original number. $\longrightarrow$ 10u+t = 5(10t+u)−9

This equation simplifies to 49t−5u = 9.

Solving the system $\begin{pmatrix} 8t - u = 0 \\ 49t-5u = 9 \end{pmatrix}$ produces t = 1 and u = 8. Therefore, the number is 18.

57. Let ℓ represent the length and w the width.

If the width is increased by 2 and the
length is not changed, the area is
increased by 36. $\longrightarrow$ ℓ(w+2) = ℓw+36

This equation simplifies to ℓ = 18.

If the width is increased by 1 and
the length by 2, the area is
increased by 48. $\longrightarrow$ (ℓ+2)(w+1) = ℓw+48

This equation simplifies to ℓ+2w = 46.

Solving the system $\begin{pmatrix} ℓ = 18 \\ ℓ+2w = 46 \end{pmatrix}$ produces ℓ = 18 and w = 14.

1.
$$\left(\begin{array}{l} x+2y-3z = 2 \\ \quad\; 3x - z = -8 \\ 2x-3y+5z = -9 \end{array}\right) \quad \begin{array}{l} (1) \\ (2) \\ (3) \end{array}$$

Since equation (2) has no y-term, let's eliminate y from equations (1) and (3).

$$\begin{array}{ll} x+2y-3z = 2 & \underline{\text{Multiply by 3.}} \\ 2x-3y+5z = -9 & \underline{\text{Multiply by 2.}} \end{array} \quad \begin{array}{l} 3x+6y-9z = 6 \\ \underline{4x-6y+10z = -18} \\ 7x \qquad + z = -12 \end{array}$$

Now we can solve the system

$$\left(\begin{array}{l} 3x-z = -8 \\ 7x+z = -12 \end{array}\right).$$

$$\begin{array}{l} 3x-z = -8 \\ \underline{7x+z = -12} \\ 10x \quad = -20 \\ \qquad x = -2 \end{array}$$

Substitute -2 for x in $3x-z = -8$.

$$\begin{array}{l} 3(-2)-z = -8 \\ \qquad -z = -2 \\ \qquad\; z = 2 \end{array}$$

Substitute -2 for x and 2 for z in equation (1).

$$\begin{array}{l} x+2y-3z = 2 \\ -2+2y-3(2) = 2 \\ \qquad 2y-8 = 2 \\ \qquad 2y = 10 \\ \qquad\; y = 5 \end{array}$$

The solution set is $\{(-2,5,2)\}$.

5.
$$\left(\begin{array}{l} 2x - y + z = 0 \\ 3x-2y +4z = 11 \\ 5x +y - 6z = -32 \end{array}\right) \quad \begin{array}{l} (1) \\ (2) \\ (3) \end{array}$$

First, let's elininate z from equations (1) and (2).

$$\begin{array}{ll} 2x - y +z = 0 & \underline{\text{Multiply by } -4.} \\ 3x-2y+4z = 11 & \underline{\text{Leave alone.}} \end{array} \quad \begin{array}{l} -8x+4y-4z = 0 \\ \underline{3x-2y+4z = 11} \\ -5x+2y \quad = 11 \end{array}$$

Now let's eliminate z from equations (1) and (3).

$$\begin{array}{ll} 2x - y +z = 0 & \underline{\text{Multiply by 6.}} \\ 5x +y-6z = -32 & \underline{\text{Leave alone.}} \end{array} \quad \begin{array}{l} 12x-6y+6z = 0 \\ \underline{5x +y-6z = -32} \\ 17x-5y \quad = -32 \end{array}$$

We now have the following system to solve.

$$\left(\begin{array}{l} -5x+2y = 11 \\ 17x-5y = -32 \end{array}\right)$$

$$\begin{array}{ll} -5x+2y = 11 & \underline{\text{Multiply by 5.}} \\ 17x-5y = -32 & \underline{\text{Multiply by 2.}} \end{array} \quad \begin{array}{l} -25x+10y = 55 \\ \underline{34x-10y = -64} \\ 9x \qquad = -9 \\ \qquad\; x = -1 \end{array}$$

Substitute -1 for x in -5x+2y = 11.

$$-5(-1)+2y = 11$$
$$2y = 6$$
$$y = 3$$

Finally, substitute -1 for x and 3 for y in equation (1).

$$2x-y+z = 0$$
$$2(-1)-3+z = 0$$
$$z = 5$$

The solution set is $\{(-1,3,5)\}$.

9. $\begin{pmatrix} x - y+2z = 4 \\ 2x-2y+4z = 7 \\ 3x-3y+6z = 1 \end{pmatrix}$ (1)
   (2)
   (3)

Let's eliminate x from equations (1) and (2).

$x - y+2z = 4$	Multiply by -2.	$-2x+2y-4z = -8$
$2x-2y+4z = 7$	Leave alone.	$2x-2y+4z = 7$
		$0 = -1$

The false statement $0 = -1$ implies that the system has no solution; its solution set is $\emptyset$.

13. $\begin{pmatrix} 3x-2y+4z = 6 \\ 9x+4y - z = 0 \\ 6x-8y-3z = 3 \end{pmatrix}$ (1)
   (2)
   (3)

Let's eliminate z from equations (1) and (2).

$3x-2y+4z = 6$	Leave alone.	$3x - 2y+4z = 6$
$9x+4y - z = 0$	Multiply by 4.	$36x+16y-4z = 0$
		$39x+14y = 6$

Let's eliminate z from equations (2) and (3).

$9x+4y - z = 0$	Multiply by -3.	$-27x-12y+3z = 0$
$6x-8y-3z = 3$	Leave alone.	$6x - 8y-3z = 3$
		$-21x-20y = 3$

Now we need to solve the system

$$\begin{pmatrix} 39x+14y = 6 \\ -21x-20y = 3 \end{pmatrix}.$$

$39x+14y = 6$	Multiply by 10.	$390x+140y = 60$
$-21x-20y = 3$	Multiply by 7.	$-147x-140y = 21$
		$243x = 81$
		$x = \dfrac{1}{3}$

Substitute $\frac{1}{3}$ for x in $39x+14y = 6$.

$$39\left(\tfrac{1}{3}\right)+14y = 6$$
$$13+14y = 6$$
$$14y = -7$$
$$y = -\frac{7}{14} = -\frac{1}{2}$$

Finally, substitute $\frac{1}{3}$ for x and $-\frac{1}{2}$ for y in 3x−2y+4z = 6.

$$3\left(\frac{1}{3}\right)-2\left(-\frac{1}{2}\right)+4z = 6$$
$$1+1+4z = 6$$
$$4z = 4$$
$$z = 1$$

The solution set is $\{(\frac{1}{3},-\frac{1}{2}, 1)\}$.

17.
$$\begin{pmatrix} 4x-y+3z = -12 \\ 2x+3y-z = 8 \\ 6x+y+2z = -8 \end{pmatrix} \quad \begin{matrix}(1)\\(2)\\(3)\end{matrix}$$

Let's eliminate y from equations (1) and (2).

$$\begin{matrix} 4x-y+3z = -12 \\ 2x+3y-z = 8 \end{matrix} \quad \begin{matrix}\text{Multiply by 3.}\\ \text{Leave alone.}\end{matrix} \rightarrow \quad \begin{matrix} 12x-3y+9z = -36 \\ 2x+3y-z = 8 \\ \hline 14x \quad +8z = -28 \end{matrix}$$

Let's eliminate y from equations (2) and (3).

$$\begin{matrix} 2x+3y-z = 8 \\ 6x+y+2z = -8 \end{matrix} \quad \begin{matrix}\text{Leave alone.}\\ \text{Multiply by -3.}\end{matrix} \rightarrow \quad \begin{matrix} 2x+3y-z = 8 \\ -18x-3y-6z = 24 \\ \hline -16x \quad -7z = 32 \end{matrix}$$

The equation 14x+8z = −28 can be written as 7x+4z = −14. Now we have the following system to solve.

$$\begin{pmatrix} 7x+4z = -14 \\ -16x-7z = 32 \end{pmatrix}$$

$$\begin{matrix} 7x+4z = -14 \\ -16x-7z = 32 \end{matrix} \quad \begin{matrix}\text{Multiply by 7.}\\ \text{Multiply by 4.}\end{matrix} \rightarrow \quad \begin{matrix} 49x+28z = -98 \\ -64x-28z = 128 \\ \hline -15x \quad = 30 \\ x = -2 \end{matrix}$$

Substitute −2 for x in 7x+4z = −14.

$$7(-2)+4z = -14$$
$$4z = 0$$
$$z = 0$$

Finally, substitute −2 for x and 0 for z in 4x−y+3z = −12.

$$4(-2)-y+3(0) = -12$$
$$-y = -4$$
$$y = 4$$

The solution set is $\{(-2,4,0)\}$.

21. Let h represent the hundreds digit, t the tens digit, and u the units digit.

The sum of the digits is 14. $\longrightarrow$ $h+t+u = 14$

The number is 14 larger than
20 times the tens digit. $\longrightarrow$ $100h+10t+u = 20t+14$

The sum of the tens digit
and the units digit is 12
larger than the hundreds digit. $\longrightarrow$ $t+u = h+12$

Solving the system $\begin{pmatrix} h+t+u = 14 \\ 100h-10t+u = 14 \\ -h+t+u = 12 \end{pmatrix}$ produces h = 1, t = 9, and u = 4.

So the number is 194.

25. Let x, y, and z represent the three numbers.

The sum of the three
numbers is 20. $\longrightarrow$ $x+y+z = 20$

The sum of the first
and third numbers is
2 more than twice the
second number. $\longrightarrow$ $x + z = 2y+2$

The third number minus
the first yields three
times the second. $\longrightarrow$ $z - x = 3y$

Solving the system $\begin{pmatrix} x+y+z = 20 \\ x-2y+z = 2 \\ -x-3y+z = 0 \end{pmatrix}$ produces $x = -2$, $y = 6$, and $z = 16$.

29. Let x, y, and z represent the money invested at 12%, 13%, and 14%, respectively.

The total amount
invested is \$3000. $\longrightarrow$ $x + y + z = 3000$

The total yearly
income is \$400. $\longrightarrow$ $.12x+.13y+.14z = 400$

The sum of the amounts
invested at 12% and 13%
equals the amount in-
vested at 14%. $\longrightarrow$ $x + y = z$

Solving the system $\begin{pmatrix} x+y+z = 3000 \\ .12x + .13y + .14z = 400 \\ x+y-z = 0 \end{pmatrix}$ produces $x = 500$, $y = 1000$,
and $z = 1500$.

Problem Set 9.4

1. $\begin{pmatrix} x-2y = 14 \\ 4x+5y = 4 \end{pmatrix}$ The augmented matrix is $\begin{bmatrix} 1 & -2 & | & 14 \\ 4 & 5 & | & 4 \end{bmatrix}$.

$\begin{bmatrix} 1 & -2 & | & 14 \\ 4 & 5 & | & 4 \end{bmatrix}$ $\xrightarrow{-4(\text{Row 1}) + \text{Row 2}}$ $\begin{bmatrix} 1 & -2 & | & 14 \\ 0 & 13 & | & -52 \end{bmatrix}$

From the bottom row of the last matrix we see that $13y = -52$.

$$13y = -52$$
$$y = -4$$

Now we can substitute -4 for y in $x-2y = 14$.

$$x-2(-4) = 14$$
$$x = 6$$

The solution set is $\{(6,-4)\}$.

5. $\begin{pmatrix} x-3y = 4 \\ 4x-5y = 3 \end{pmatrix}$ The augmented matrix is $\begin{bmatrix} 1 & -3 & \vdots & 4 \\ 4 & -5 & \vdots & 3 \end{bmatrix}$.

$$\begin{bmatrix} 1 & -3 & \vdots & 4 \\ 4 & -5 & \vdots & 3 \end{bmatrix} \xrightarrow{-4(\text{Row 1}) + \text{Row 2}} \begin{bmatrix} 1 & -3 & \vdots & 4 \\ 0 & 7 & \vdots & -13 \end{bmatrix}$$

From the bottom row of the last matrix we obtain $7y = -13$.

$$7y = -13$$
$$y = -\frac{13}{7}$$

Now we can substitute $-\frac{13}{7}$ for y in $x-3y = 4$.

$$x - 3\left(-\frac{13}{7}\right) = 4$$
$$x + \frac{39}{7} = 4$$
$$x = -\frac{11}{7}$$

The solution set is $\left\{\left(-\frac{11}{7}, -\frac{13}{7}\right)\right\}$.

9. $\begin{pmatrix} x+3y-4z = 5 \\ -2x-5y+z = 9 \\ 7x-y-z = -2 \end{pmatrix}$ We can work with the augmented matrix as follows.

$$\begin{bmatrix} 1 & 3 & -4 & \vdots & 5 \\ -2 & -5 & 1 & \vdots & 9 \\ 7 & -1 & -1 & \vdots & -2 \end{bmatrix} \begin{array}{c} \xrightarrow{2(\text{Row 1}) + \text{Row 2}} \\ \xrightarrow{-7(\text{Row 1}) + \text{Row 3}} \end{array} \begin{bmatrix} 1 & 3 & -4 & \vdots & 5 \\ 0 & 1 & -7 & \vdots & 19 \\ 0 & -22 & 27 & \vdots & -37 \end{bmatrix}$$

$$\begin{bmatrix} 1 & 3 & -4 & \vdots & 5 \\ 0 & 1 & -7 & \vdots & 19 \\ 0 & -22 & 27 & \vdots & -37 \end{bmatrix} \xrightarrow{22(\text{Row 2}) + \text{Row 3}} \begin{bmatrix} 1 & 3 & -4 & \vdots & 5 \\ 0 & 1 & -7 & \vdots & 19 \\ 0 & 0 & -127 & \vdots & 381 \end{bmatrix}$$

The last matrix represents the system

$$\begin{pmatrix} x+3y-4z = 5 \\ y-7z = 19 \\ -127z = 381 \end{pmatrix}. \quad \begin{array}{c} (1) \\ (2) \\ (3) \end{array}$$

From equation (3) we obtain

$$-127z = 381$$
$$z = -3.$$

Substitute -3 for z in equation (2).

$$y-7(-3) = 19$$
$$y = -2$$

Finally, substitute -3 for z and -2 for y in equation (1).

$$x+3(-2)-4(-3) = 5$$
$$x-6+12 = 5$$
$$x = -1$$

The solution set is $\{(-1,-2,-3)\}$.

13. $\begin{pmatrix} y + 3z = -3 \\ 2x - 5z = 18 \\ 3x - y + 2z = 5 \end{pmatrix}$ We can work with the augmented matrix as follows.

$$\left[\begin{array}{ccc|c} 0 & 1 & 3 & -3 \\ 2 & 0 & -5 & 18 \\ 3 & -1 & 2 & 5 \end{array}\right] \quad \begin{array}{c}\text{Exchange} \\ \text{Rows 1 and 2}\end{array} \quad \left[\begin{array}{ccc|c} 2 & 0 & -5 & 18 \\ 0 & 1 & 3 & -3 \\ 3 & -1 & 2 & 5 \end{array}\right]$$

$$\left[\begin{array}{ccc|c} 2 & 0 & -5 & 18 \\ 0 & 1 & 3 & -3 \\ 3 & -1 & 2 & 5 \end{array}\right] \quad \xrightarrow{\frac{1}{2}(\text{Row 1})} \quad \left[\begin{array}{ccc|c} 1 & 0 & -\frac{5}{2} & 9 \\ 0 & 1 & 3 & -3 \\ 3 & -1 & 2 & 5 \end{array}\right]$$

$$\left[\begin{array}{ccc|c} 1 & 0 & -\frac{5}{2} & 9 \\ 0 & 1 & 3 & -3 \\ 3 & -1 & 2 & 5 \end{array}\right] \quad \xrightarrow{-3(\text{Row 1}) + \text{Row 3}} \quad \left[\begin{array}{ccc|c} 1 & 0 & -\frac{5}{2} & 9 \\ 0 & 1 & 3 & -3 \\ 0 & -1 & \frac{19}{2} & -22 \end{array}\right]$$

$$\left[\begin{array}{ccc|c} 1 & 0 & -\frac{5}{2} & 9 \\ 0 & 1 & 3 & -3 \\ 0 & -1 & \frac{19}{2} & -22 \end{array}\right] \quad \xrightarrow{\text{Row 2} + \text{Row 3}} \quad \left[\begin{array}{ccc|c} 1 & 0 & -\frac{5}{2} & 9 \\ 0 & 1 & 3 & -3 \\ 0 & 0 & \frac{25}{2} & -25 \end{array}\right]$$

The last matrix represents the system

$$\begin{pmatrix} x - \frac{5}{2}z = 9 \\ y + 3z = -3 \\ \frac{25}{2}z = -25 \end{pmatrix}. \qquad \begin{array}{c}(1) \\ (2) \\ (3)\end{array}$$

From equation (3) we obtain

$$\frac{25}{2}z = -25$$
$$z = -2.$$

Substitute -2 for z in equation (2).

$$y + 3(-2) = -3$$
$$y = 3$$

Finally, substitute -2 for z in equation (1).

$$x - \frac{5}{2}(-2) = 9$$
$$x = 4$$

The solution set is $\{(4,3,-2)\}$.

17. $\begin{pmatrix} x+2y-z = -5 \\ 3x+4y+2z = -8 \\ -2x-y+5z = 10 \end{pmatrix}$ We can work with the augmented matrix as follows.

$$\left[\begin{array}{ccc|c} 1 & 2 & -1 & -5 \\ 3 & 4 & 2 & -8 \\ -2 & -1 & 5 & 10 \end{array}\right] \xrightarrow[\ 2(\text{Row 1})+\text{Row 3}\ ]{-3(\text{Row 1})+\text{Row 2}} \left[\begin{array}{ccc|c} 1 & 2 & -1 & -5 \\ 0 & -2 & 5 & 7 \\ 0 & 3 & 3 & 0 \end{array}\right]$$

$$\left[\begin{array}{ccc|c} 1 & 2 & -1 & -5 \\ 0 & -2 & 5 & 7 \\ 0 & 3 & 3 & 0 \end{array}\right] \xrightarrow[\ \frac{1}{3}(\text{Row 3})\ ]{-\frac{1}{2}(\text{Row 2})} \left[\begin{array}{ccc|c} 1 & 2 & -1 & -5 \\ 0 & 1 & -\frac{5}{2} & -\frac{7}{2} \\ 0 & 1 & 1 & 0 \end{array}\right]$$

$$\left[\begin{array}{ccc|c} 1 & 2 & -1 & -5 \\ 0 & 1 & -\frac{5}{2} & -\frac{7}{2} \\ 0 & 1 & 1 & 0 \end{array}\right] \xrightarrow{-1(\text{Row 2})+\text{Row 3}} \left[\begin{array}{ccc|c} 1 & 2 & -1 & -5 \\ 0 & 1 & -\frac{5}{2} & -\frac{7}{2} \\ 0 & 0 & \frac{7}{2} & \frac{7}{2} \end{array}\right]$$

The last matrix represents the system $\begin{pmatrix} x+2y-z = -5 & (1) \\ y-\frac{5}{2}z = -\frac{7}{2} & (2) \\ \frac{7}{2}z = \frac{7}{2} & (3) \end{pmatrix}$.

From equation (3) we obtain

$$\frac{7}{2}z = \frac{7}{2}$$
$$z = 1.$$

Now we can substitute 1 for z in equation (2).

$$y - \frac{5}{2}(1) = -\frac{7}{2}$$
$$y = -1$$

Finally, we can substitute 1 for z and −1 for y in equation (1).

$$x+2(-1)-(1) = -5$$
$$x-3 = -5$$
$$x = -2$$

The solution set is $\{(-2,-1,1)\}$.

21. $\begin{pmatrix} -2x+5y-z = -1 \\ 4x+y-5z = 23 \\ x-2y+3z = -7 \end{pmatrix}$ We can work with the augmented matrix as follows.

$$\left[\begin{array}{ccc|c} -2 & 5 & -1 & -1 \\ 4 & 1 & -5 & 23 \\ 1 & -2 & 3 & -7 \end{array}\right] \begin{array}{l} \text{Exchange} \\ \text{Row 1 and} \\ \text{Row 3.} \end{array} \left[\begin{array}{ccc|c} 1 & -2 & 3 & -7 \\ 4 & 1 & -5 & 23 \\ -2 & 5 & -1 & -1 \end{array}\right]$$

$$\begin{bmatrix} 1 & -2 & 3 & \vdots & -7 \\ 4 & 1 & -5 & \vdots & 23 \\ -2 & 5 & -1 & \vdots & -1 \end{bmatrix} \xrightarrow[\;2(\text{Row } 1)+\text{Row } 3\;]{-4(\text{Row } 1)+\text{Row } 2} \begin{bmatrix} 1 & -2 & 3 & \vdots & -7 \\ 0 & 9 & -17 & \vdots & 51 \\ 0 & 1 & 5 & \vdots & -15 \end{bmatrix}$$

$$\begin{bmatrix} 1 & -2 & 3 & \vdots & -7 \\ 0 & 9 & -17 & \vdots & 51 \\ 0 & 1 & 5 & \vdots & -15 \end{bmatrix} \begin{array}{c} \text{Exchange} \\ \text{Row 2 and} \\ \text{Row 3.} \end{array} \begin{bmatrix} 1 & -2 & 3 & \vdots & -7 \\ 0 & 1 & 5 & \vdots & -15 \\ 0 & 9 & -17 & \vdots & 51 \end{bmatrix}$$

$$\begin{bmatrix} 1 & -2 & 3 & \vdots & -7 \\ 0 & 1 & 5 & \vdots & -15 \\ 0 & 9 & -17 & \vdots & 51 \end{bmatrix} \xrightarrow{-9(\text{Row } 2)+\text{Row } 3} \begin{bmatrix} 1 & -2 & 3 & \vdots & -7 \\ 0 & 1 & 5 & \vdots & -15 \\ 0 & 0 & -62 & \vdots & 186 \end{bmatrix}$$

The last matrix represents the system
$$\begin{pmatrix} x-2y+3z & = & -7 \\ y+5z & = & -15 \\ -62z & = & 186 \end{pmatrix}. \qquad \begin{array}{l} (1) \\ (2) \\ (3) \end{array}$$

From equation (3) we obtain
$$-62z = 186$$
$$z = -3.$$

Now we can substitute -3 for z in equation (2).
$$y+5(-3) = -15$$
$$y = 0$$

Finally, we can substitute -3 for z and 0 for y in equation (1).
$$x-2(0)+3(-3) = -7$$
$$x = 2$$

The solution set is $\{(2,0,-3)\}$.

Problem Set 9.5

1. $\begin{vmatrix} 6 & 2 \\ 4 & 3 \end{vmatrix} = 6(3)-2(4) = 18-8 = 10$

5. $\begin{vmatrix} -3 & 2 \\ 7 & 5 \end{vmatrix} = -3(5)-2(7) = -15-14 = -29$

9. $\begin{vmatrix} -3 & 2 \\ 5 & -6 \end{vmatrix} = -3(-6)-2(5) = 18-10 = 8$

13. $\begin{vmatrix} -7 & -2 \\ -2 & 4 \end{vmatrix} = -7(4)-(-2)(-2) = -28-4 = -32$

17. $\begin{vmatrix} \frac{1}{4} & -2 \\ \frac{3}{2} & 8 \end{vmatrix} = \frac{1}{4}(8)-(-2)\left(\frac{3}{2}\right) = 2+3 = 5$

21. $\begin{pmatrix} 2x+y = 14 \\ 3x-y = 1 \end{pmatrix}$

$$D = \begin{vmatrix} 2 & 1 \\ 3 & -1 \end{vmatrix} = 2(-1)-1(3) = -2-3 = -5$$

$$D_x = \begin{vmatrix} 14 & 1 \\ 1 & -1 \end{vmatrix} = 14(-1)-1(1) = -14-1 = -15$$

$$D_y = \begin{vmatrix} 2 & 14 \\ 3 & 1 \end{vmatrix} = 2(1)-14(3) = 2-42 = -40$$

$$x = \frac{D_x}{D} = \frac{-15}{-5} = 3 \text{ and } y = \frac{D_y}{D} = \frac{-40}{-5} = 8$$

The solution set is $\{(3,8)\}$.

25. $\begin{pmatrix} 9x+5y = -8 \\ 7x-4y = -22 \end{pmatrix}$

$$D = \begin{vmatrix} 9 & 5 \\ 7 & -4 \end{vmatrix} = 9(-4)-5(7) = -36-35 = -71$$

$$D_x = \begin{vmatrix} -8 & 5 \\ -22 & -4 \end{vmatrix} = -8(-4)-5(-22) = 32+110 = 142$$

$$D_y = \begin{vmatrix} 9 & -8 \\ 7 & -22 \end{vmatrix} = 9(-22)-(-8)(7) = -198+56 = -142$$

$$x = \frac{D_x}{D} = \frac{142}{-71} = -2 \text{ and } y = \frac{D_y}{D} = \frac{-142}{-71} = 2$$

The solution set is $\{(-2,2)\}$.

29. $\begin{pmatrix} 6x - y = 0 \\ 5x+4y = 29 \end{pmatrix}$

$$D = \begin{vmatrix} 6 & -1 \\ 5 & 4 \end{vmatrix} = 6(4)-(-1)(5) = 24+5 = 29$$

$$D_x = \begin{vmatrix} 0 & -1 \\ 29 & 4 \end{vmatrix} = 0(4)-(-1)(29) = 0+29 = 29$$

$$D_y = \begin{vmatrix} 6 & 0 \\ 4 & 29 \end{vmatrix} = 6(29)-(0)(5) = 174-0 = 174$$

$$x = \frac{D_x}{D} = \frac{29}{29} = 1 \text{ and } y = \frac{D_y}{D} = \frac{174}{29} = 6$$

The solution set is $\{(1,6)\}$.

33. $\begin{pmatrix} 6x-5y & = & 1 \\ 4x+7y & = & 2 \end{pmatrix}$

$$D = \begin{vmatrix} 6 & -5 \\ 4 & 7 \end{vmatrix} = 6(7)-(-5)(4) = 42+20 = 62$$

$$D_x = \begin{vmatrix} 1 & -5 \\ 2 & 7 \end{vmatrix} = 1(7)-(-5)(2) = 7+10 = 17$$

$$D_y = \begin{vmatrix} 6 & 1 \\ 4 & 2 \end{vmatrix} = 6(2)-1(4) = 12-4 = 8$$

$$x = \frac{D_x}{D} = \frac{17}{62} \quad \text{and} \quad y = \frac{D_y}{D} = \frac{8}{62} = \frac{4}{31}$$

The solution set is $\{(\frac{17}{62},\frac{4}{31})\}$.

37. $\begin{pmatrix} -\frac{2}{3}x + \frac{1}{2}y & = & -7 \\ \frac{1}{3}x - \frac{3}{2}y & = & 6 \end{pmatrix}$

$$D = \begin{vmatrix} -\frac{2}{3} & \frac{1}{2} \\ \frac{1}{3} & -\frac{3}{2} \end{vmatrix} = -\frac{2}{3}(-\frac{3}{2}) - \frac{1}{2}(\frac{1}{3}) = 1 - \frac{1}{6} = \frac{5}{6}$$

$$D_x = \begin{vmatrix} -7 & \frac{1}{2} \\ 6 & -\frac{3}{2} \end{vmatrix} = -7(-\frac{3}{2}) - \frac{1}{2}(6) = \frac{21}{2} - 3 = \frac{15}{2}$$

$$D_y = \begin{vmatrix} -\frac{2}{3} & -7 \\ \frac{1}{3} & 6 \end{vmatrix} = -\frac{2}{3}(6)-(-7)(\frac{1}{3}) = -4 + \frac{7}{3} = -\frac{5}{3}$$

$$x = \frac{D_x}{D} = \frac{\frac{15}{2}}{\frac{5}{6}} = 9 \quad \text{and} \quad y = \frac{D_y}{D} = \frac{-\frac{5}{3}}{\frac{5}{6}} = -2$$

The solution set is $\{(9,-2)\}$.

[You may wish to clear the original equations of fractions first and then use Cramer's Rule.]

Problem Set 9.6

1. Let's expand by minors about the first column.

$$\begin{vmatrix} 2 & 7 & 5 \\ 1 & -1 & 1 \\ -4 & 3 & 2 \end{vmatrix} = 2\begin{vmatrix} -1 & 1 \\ 3 & 2 \end{vmatrix} - 1\begin{vmatrix} 7 & 5 \\ 3 & 2 \end{vmatrix} - 4\begin{vmatrix} 7 & 5 \\ -1 & 1 \end{vmatrix}$$

$$= 2(-2-3)-1(14-15)-4(7+5) = 2(-5)-1(-1)-4(12) = -10+1-48 = -57$$

5. Let's expand about the 2nd column.

$$\begin{vmatrix} -3 & -2 & 1 \\ 5 & 0 & 6 \\ 2 & 1 & -4 \end{vmatrix} = -(-2)\begin{vmatrix} 5 & 6 \\ 2 & -4 \end{vmatrix} + 0\begin{vmatrix} -3 & 1 \\ 2 & -4 \end{vmatrix} - 1\begin{vmatrix} -3 & 1 \\ 5 & 6 \end{vmatrix}$$

$$= 2(-32)+0-1(-23) = -41$$

9. Let's expand about the first column.

$$\begin{vmatrix} 4 & -2 & 7 \\ 1 & -1 & 6 \\ 3 & 5 & -2 \end{vmatrix} = 4\begin{vmatrix} -1 & 6 \\ 5 & -2 \end{vmatrix} - 1\begin{vmatrix} -2 & 7 \\ 5 & -2 \end{vmatrix} + 3\begin{vmatrix} -2 & 7 \\ -1 & 6 \end{vmatrix}$$

$$= 4(-28)-1(-31)+3(-5) = -112+31-15 = -96$$

13. $$\begin{pmatrix} x - y +2z = -8 \\ 2x+3y-4z = 18 \\ -x+2y - z = 7 \end{pmatrix}$$

$$D = \begin{vmatrix} 1 & -1 & 2 \\ 2 & 3 & -4 \\ -1 & 2 & -1 \end{vmatrix} = 1\begin{vmatrix} 3 & -4 \\ 2 & -1 \end{vmatrix} - 2\begin{vmatrix} -1 & 2 \\ 2 & -1 \end{vmatrix} - 1\begin{vmatrix} -1 & 2 \\ 3 & -4 \end{vmatrix}$$

(Expand about $\quad = 1(5)-2(-3)-1(-2) = 5+6+2 = 13$
1st column.)

$$D_x = \begin{vmatrix} -8 & -1 & 2 \\ 18 & 3 & -4 \\ 7 & 2 & -1 \end{vmatrix} = -8\begin{vmatrix} 3 & -4 \\ 2 & -1 \end{vmatrix} - 18\begin{vmatrix} -1 & 2 \\ 2 & -1 \end{vmatrix} + 7\begin{vmatrix} -1 & 2 \\ 3 & -4 \end{vmatrix}$$

(Expand about $\quad = -8(5)-18(-3)+7(-2) = -40+54-14 = 0$
1st column.)

$$D_y = \begin{vmatrix} 1 & -8 & 2 \\ 2 & 18 & -4 \\ -1 & 7 & -1 \end{vmatrix} = -(-8)\begin{vmatrix} 2 & -4 \\ -1 & -1 \end{vmatrix} + 18\begin{vmatrix} 1 & 2 \\ -1 & -1 \end{vmatrix} - 7\begin{vmatrix} 1 & 2 \\ 2 & -4 \end{vmatrix}$$

(Expand about $\quad = 8(-6)+18(1)-7(-8) = -48+18+56 = 26$
2nd column.)

$$D_z = \begin{vmatrix} 1 & -1 & -8 \\ 2 & 3 & 18 \\ -1 & 2 & 7 \end{vmatrix} = -8\begin{vmatrix} 2 & 3 \\ -1 & 2 \end{vmatrix} - 18\begin{vmatrix} 1 & -1 \\ -1 & 2 \end{vmatrix} + 7\begin{vmatrix} 1 & -1 \\ 2 & 3 \end{vmatrix}$$

(Expand about $\quad$ $= -8(7)-18(1)+7(5) = -56-18+35 = -39$
3rd column.

$$x = \frac{D_x}{D} = \frac{0}{13} = 0, \quad y = \frac{D_y}{D} = \frac{26}{13} = 2, \quad z = \frac{D_z}{D} = \frac{-39}{13} = -3$$

The solution set is $\{(0,2,-3)\}$.

17. $\begin{pmatrix} -x + y + z = -1 \\ x-2y+5z = -4 \\ 3x+4y-6z = -1 \end{pmatrix}$

$$D = \begin{vmatrix} -1 & 1 & 1 \\ 1 & -2 & 5 \\ 3 & 4 & -6 \end{vmatrix} = -1\begin{vmatrix} -2 & 5 \\ 4 & -6 \end{vmatrix} - 1\begin{vmatrix} 1 & 1 \\ 4 & -6 \end{vmatrix} + 3\begin{vmatrix} 1 & 1 \\ -2 & 5 \end{vmatrix}$$

(Expand about $\quad$ $= -1(-8)-1(-10)+3(7) = 8+10+21 = 39$
1st column.)

$$D_x = \begin{vmatrix} -1 & 1 & 1 \\ -4 & -2 & 5 \\ -1 & 4 & -6 \end{vmatrix} = -1\begin{vmatrix} -2 & 5 \\ 4 & -6 \end{vmatrix} - (-4)\begin{vmatrix} 1 & 1 \\ 4 & -6 \end{vmatrix} - 1\begin{vmatrix} 1 & 1 \\ -2 & 5 \end{vmatrix}$$

(Expand about $\quad$ $= -1(-8)+4(-10)-1(7) = 8-40-7 = -39$
1st column.)

$$D_y = \begin{vmatrix} -1 & -1 & 1 \\ 1 & -4 & 5 \\ 3 & -1 & -6 \end{vmatrix} = -1\begin{vmatrix} -4 & 5 \\ -1 & -6 \end{vmatrix} - 1\begin{vmatrix} -1 & 1 \\ -1 & -6 \end{vmatrix} + 3\begin{vmatrix} -1 & 1 \\ -4 & 5 \end{vmatrix}$$

(Expand about $\quad$ $= -1(29)-1(7)+3(-1) = -29-7-3 = -39$
1st column.)

$$D_z = \begin{vmatrix} -1 & 1 & -1 \\ 1 & -2 & -4 \\ 3 & 4 & -1 \end{vmatrix} = -1\begin{vmatrix} -2 & -4 \\ 4 & -1 \end{vmatrix} - 1\begin{vmatrix} 1 & -1 \\ 4 & -1 \end{vmatrix} + 3\begin{vmatrix} 1 & -1 \\ -2 & -4 \end{vmatrix}$$

(Expand about $\quad$ $= -1(18)-1(3)+3(-6) = -18-3-18 = -39$
1st column.)

$$x = \frac{D_x}{D} = \frac{-39}{39} = -1, \quad y = \frac{D_y}{D} = \frac{-39}{39} = -1, \quad z = \frac{D_z}{D} = \frac{-39}{39} = -1$$

The solution set is $\{(-1,-1,-1)\}$.

21. $\begin{pmatrix} 2x - y+3z & = & -5 \\ 3x+4y-2z & = & -25 \\ -x+z & = & 6 \end{pmatrix}$

$$D = \begin{vmatrix} 2 & -1 & 3 \\ 3 & 4 & -2 \\ -1 & 0 & 1 \end{vmatrix} = -1(-1)\begin{vmatrix} 3 & -2 \\ -1 & 1 \end{vmatrix} + 4\begin{vmatrix} 2 & 3 \\ -1 & 1 \end{vmatrix} - 0\begin{vmatrix} 2 & 3 \\ 3 & -2 \end{vmatrix}$$

(Expand about 2nd column.)
$$= 1(1)+4(5)-0 = 21$$

$$D_x = \begin{vmatrix} -5 & -1 & 3 \\ -25 & 4 & -2 \\ 6 & 0 & 1 \end{vmatrix} = -5\begin{vmatrix} 4 & -2 \\ 0 & 1 \end{vmatrix} - (-25)\begin{vmatrix} -1 & 3 \\ 0 & 1 \end{vmatrix} + 6\begin{vmatrix} -1 & 3 \\ 4 & -2 \end{vmatrix}$$

(Expand about 1st column.)
$$= -5(4)+25(-1)+6(-10) = -20-25-60 = -105$$

$$D_y = \begin{vmatrix} 2 & -5 & 3 \\ 3 & -25 & -2 \\ -1 & 6 & 1 \end{vmatrix} = -(-5)\begin{vmatrix} 3 & -2 \\ -1 & 1 \end{vmatrix} - 25\begin{vmatrix} 2 & 3 \\ -1 & 1 \end{vmatrix} - 6\begin{vmatrix} 2 & 3 \\ 3 & -2 \end{vmatrix}$$

(Expand about 2nd column.)
$$= 5(1)-25(5)-6(-13) = 5-125+78 = -42$$

$$D_z = \begin{vmatrix} 2 & -1 & -5 \\ 3 & 4 & -25 \\ -1 & 0 & 6 \end{vmatrix} = -(-1)\begin{vmatrix} 3 & -25 \\ -1 & 6 \end{vmatrix} + 4\begin{vmatrix} 2 & -5 \\ -1 & 6 \end{vmatrix} - 0\begin{vmatrix} 2 & -5 \\ 3 & -25 \end{vmatrix}$$

(Expand about 2nd column.
$$= 1(-7)+4(7)-0 = -7+28 = 21$$

$$x = \frac{D_x}{D} = \frac{-105}{21} = -5, \quad y = \frac{D_y}{D} = \frac{-42}{21} = -2, \quad z = \frac{D_z}{D} = \frac{21}{21} = 1$$

The solution set is $\{(-5,-2,1)\}$.

25. $\begin{pmatrix} -2x+5y-3z & = & -1 \\ 2x-7y+3z & = & 1 \\ 4x-y-6z & = & -6 \end{pmatrix}$

$$D = \begin{vmatrix} -2 & 5 & -3 \\ 2 & -7 & 3 \\ 4 & -1 & -6 \end{vmatrix} = -2\begin{vmatrix} -7 & 3 \\ -1 & -6 \end{vmatrix} - 2\begin{vmatrix} 5 & -3 \\ -1 & -6 \end{vmatrix} + 4\begin{vmatrix} 5 & -3 \\ -7 & 3 \end{vmatrix}$$

(Expand about 1st column.)
$$= -2(45)-2(-33)+4(-6) = -90+66-24 = -48$$

$$D_x = \begin{vmatrix} -1 & 5 & -3 \\ 1 & -7 & 3 \\ -6 & -1 & -6 \end{vmatrix} = -1\begin{vmatrix} -7 & 3 \\ -1 & -6 \end{vmatrix} - 1\begin{vmatrix} 5 & -3 \\ -1 & -6 \end{vmatrix} - 6\begin{vmatrix} 5 & -3 \\ -7 & 3 \end{vmatrix}$$

(Expand about 1st column.)
$$= -1(45)-1(-33)-6(-6) = -45+33+36 = 24$$

$$D_y = \begin{vmatrix} -2 & -1 & -3 \\ 2 & 1 & 3 \\ 4 & -6 & -6 \end{vmatrix} = -2\begin{vmatrix} 1 & 3 \\ -6 & -6 \end{vmatrix} - 2\begin{vmatrix} -1 & -3 \\ -6 & -6 \end{vmatrix} + 4\begin{vmatrix} -1 & -3 \\ 1 & 3 \end{vmatrix}$$

$$= -2(12)-2(-12)+4(0) = -24+24+0 = 0$$

$$D_z = \begin{vmatrix} -2 & 5 & -1 \\ 2 & -7 & 1 \\ 4 & -1 & -6 \end{vmatrix} = -2\begin{vmatrix} -7 & 1 \\ -1 & -6 \end{vmatrix} - 2\begin{vmatrix} 5 & -1 \\ -1 & -6 \end{vmatrix} + 4\begin{vmatrix} 5 & -1 \\ -7 & 1 \end{vmatrix}$$

$$= -2(43)-2(-31)+4(-2)= -86+62-8 = -32$$

$$x = \frac{D_x}{D} = \frac{24}{-48} = -\frac{1}{2}, \quad y = \frac{D_y}{D} = \frac{0}{-48} = 0, \quad z = \frac{D_z}{D} = \frac{-32}{-48} = \frac{2}{3}$$

The solution set is $\{(-\frac{1}{2}, 0, \frac{2}{3})\}$.

29. $\begin{pmatrix} 5x - y+2z = 10 \\ 7x+2y-2z = -4 \\ -3x - y+4z = 1 \end{pmatrix}$

$$D = \begin{vmatrix} 5 & -1 & 2 \\ 7 & 2 & -2 \\ -3 & -1 & 4 \end{vmatrix} = 5\begin{vmatrix} 2 & -2 \\ -1 & 4 \end{vmatrix} - 7\begin{vmatrix} -1 & 2 \\ -1 & 4 \end{vmatrix} - 3\begin{vmatrix} -1 & 2 \\ 2 & -2 \end{vmatrix}$$

(Expand about 1st column.)

$$= 5(6)-7(-2)-3(-2) = 30+14+6 = 50$$

$$D_x = \begin{vmatrix} 10 & -1 & 2 \\ -4 & 2 & -2 \\ 1 & -1 & 4 \end{vmatrix} = 10\begin{vmatrix} 2 & -2 \\ -1 & 4 \end{vmatrix} + 4\begin{vmatrix} -1 & 2 \\ -1 & 4 \end{vmatrix} + 1\begin{vmatrix} -1 & 2 \\ 2 & -2 \end{vmatrix}$$

(Expand about 1st column.)

$$= 10(6)+4(-2)+1(-2) = 60-8-2 = 50$$

$$D_y = \begin{vmatrix} 5 & 10 & 2 \\ 7 & -4 & -2 \\ -3 & 1 & 4 \end{vmatrix} = 5\begin{vmatrix} -4 & -2 \\ 1 & 4 \end{vmatrix} - 7\begin{vmatrix} 10 & 2 \\ 1 & 4 \end{vmatrix} - 3\begin{vmatrix} 10 & 2 \\ -4 & -2 \end{vmatrix}$$

(Expand about 1st column.)

$$= 5(-14)-7(38)-3(-12) = -70-266+36 = -300$$

$$D_z = \begin{vmatrix} 5 & -1 & 10 \\ 7 & 2 & -4 \\ -3 & -1 & 1 \end{vmatrix} = 5\begin{vmatrix} 2 & -4 \\ -1 & 1 \end{vmatrix} - 7\begin{vmatrix} -1 & 10 \\ -1 & 1 \end{vmatrix} - 3\begin{vmatrix} -1 & 10 \\ 2 & -4 \end{vmatrix}$$

$$= 5(-2)-7(9)-3(-16) = -10-63+48 = -25$$

$$x = \frac{D_x}{D} = \frac{50}{50} = 1, \quad y = \frac{D_y}{D} = \frac{-300}{50} = -6, \quad z = \frac{D_z}{D} = \frac{-25}{50} = -\frac{1}{2}$$

The solution set is $\{(1,-6, -\frac{1}{2})\}$.

1. $\left(\begin{array}{l} y = (x+2)^2 \\ y = -2x-4 \end{array}\right)$ We can equate the values of y.

$$(x+2)^2 = -2x-4$$
$$x^2+4x+4 = -2x-4$$
$$x^2+6x+8 = 0$$
$$(x+4)(x+2) = 0$$
$$x+4 = 0 \quad \text{or} \quad x+2 = 0$$
$$x = -4 \quad \text{or} \quad x = -2$$

Substitute -4 for x in y = -2x-4.

$$y = -2(-4)-4 = 8-4 = 4$$

Therefore, (-4,4) is a solution.

Substitute -2 for x in y = -2x-4.

$$y = -2(-2)-4 = 4-4 = 0$$

Therefore, (-2,0) is a solution.

The solution set is $\{(-2,0),(-4,4)\}$.

5. $\left(\begin{array}{l} y = x^2+6x+7 \\ 2x+y = -5 \end{array}\right)$

From the first equation we can substitute x^2+6x+7 for y in the second equation.

$$2x+x^2+6x+7 = -5$$
$$x^2+8x+12 = 0$$
$$(x+6)(x+2) = 0$$
$$x+6 = 0 \quad \text{or} \quad x+2 = 0$$
$$x = -6 \quad \text{or} \quad x = -2$$

Substitute -6 for x in 2x+y = -5.

$$2(-6)+y = -5$$
$$-12+y = -5$$
$$y = 7$$

Therefore, (-6,7) is a solution.

Substitute -2 for x in 2x+y = -5.

$$2(-2)+y = -5$$
$$-4+y = -5$$
$$y = -1$$

Therefore, (-2,-1) is a solution.

The solution set is $\{(-6,7),(-2,-1)\}$.

9. $\left(\begin{array}{l} x+y = -8 \\ x^2-y^2 = 16 \end{array}\right)$ The first equation can be written as y = -x-8.

Substitute -x-8 for y in the second equation.

$$x^2-(-x-8)^2 = 16$$
$$x^2-(x^2+16x+64) = 16$$
$$x^2-x^2-16x-64 = 16$$
$$-16x = 80$$
$$x = -5$$

Substitute -5 for x in x+y = -8.

$$-5+y = -8$$
$$y = -3$$

The solution set is $\{(-5,-3)\}$.

13. $\left(\begin{array}{l} xy = 4 \\ y = x \end{array}\right)$

From the second equation we can substitute x for y in the first equation.

$$x(x) = 4$$
$$x^2 = 4$$
$$x = \pm 2$$

The solution set is $\{(2,2),(-2,-2)\}$.

Chapter 10

Problem Set 10.1

1. $3^x = 27$

   $3^x = 3^3$

   $x = 3$

   The solution set is $\{3\}$.

5. $(\frac{1}{4})^x = \frac{1}{256}$

   $(\frac{1}{4})^x = (\frac{1}{4})^4$

   $x = 4$

   The solution set is $\{4\}$.

9. $3^{-x} = \frac{1}{243}$

   $3^{-x} = \frac{1}{3^5}$

   $3^{-x} = 3^{-5}$

   $-x = -5$

   $x = 5$

   The solution set is $\{5\}$.

13. $4^x = 8$

    $(2^2)^x = 2^3$

    $2^{2x} = 2^3$

    $2x = 3$

    $x = \frac{3}{2}$

    The solution set is $\{\frac{3}{2}\}$.

17. $(\frac{1}{2})^{2x} = 64$

    $(2^{-1})^{2x} = 2^6$

    $2^{-2x} = 2^6$

    $-2x = 6$

    $x = -3$

    The solution set is $\{-3\}$.

21. $9^{4x-2} = \frac{1}{81}$

    $(3^2)^{4x-2} = \frac{1}{3^4}$

    $3^{8x-4} = 3^{-4}$

    $8x-4 = -4$

    $8x = 0$

    $x = 0$

    The solution set is $\{0\}$.

25. $10^x = .1$

    $10^x = \frac{1}{10}$

    $10^x = 10^{-1}$

    $x = -1$

    The solution set is $\{-1\}$.

29. $(2^{x+1})(2^x) = 64$

    $2^{x+1+x} = 2^6$

    $2^{x+1} = 2^6$

    $2x+1 = 6$

    $2x = 5$

    $x = \frac{5}{2}$

    The solution set is $\{\frac{5}{2}\}$.

33. $\quad (4^x)(16^{3x-1}) = 8$

$\qquad (2^2)^x (2^4)^{3x-1} = 2^3$

$\qquad (2^{2x})(2^{12x-4}) = 2^3$

$\qquad\qquad 2^{2x+12x-4} = 2^3$

$\qquad\qquad\quad 2^{14x-4} = 2^3$

$\qquad\qquad\quad 14x-4 = 3$

$\qquad\qquad\qquad 14x = 7$

$\qquad\qquad\qquad\quad x = \dfrac{7}{14} = \dfrac{1}{2}$

The solution set is $\{\frac{1}{2}\}$.

37. $\quad f(x) = 6^x$

The points $(0,1), (1,6),$ and $(-1,\frac{1}{6})$ along with the knowledge of the general shape of an exponential curve should allow you to sketch this curve.

41. $\quad f(x) = (\frac{3}{4})^x$

The points $(-1,\frac{4}{3}), (0,1),$ and $(1,\frac{3}{4})$ along with the knowledge of the general shape of an exponential curve should allow you to sketch this curve.

45. $\quad f(x) = 3^{-x}$

This curve is a vertical axis reflection of $f(x) = 3^x$. You can also graph it by plotting a few points such as $(-1,3), (0,1),$ and $(1,\frac{1}{3})$.

49. $\quad f(x) = 3^x - 2$

This is the graph of $f(x) = 3^x$ shifted down two units.

Problem Set 10.2

1. (a) $\quad P = P_0(1.04)^t = .55(1.04)^3 = .62$

   (e) $\quad P = P_0(1.04)^t = 9000(1.04)^5 = 10949.88$

5. $\quad A = P(1 + \frac{r}{n})^{nt} = 500(1 + \frac{.08}{2})^{2(7)} = 500(1.04)^{14} = \$865.84$

9. $\quad A = P(1 + \frac{r}{n})^{nt} = 1500(1 + \frac{.12}{12})^{12(5)} = 1500(1.01)^{60} = \$2725.04$

13. $\quad A = P(1 + \frac{r}{n})^{nt} = 8000(1 + \frac{.105}{4})^{4(10)} = 8000(1.02625)^{40} = \$22553.65$

17. $\quad A = Pe^{rt} = 750(2.718)^{(.08)(8)} = 750(2.718)^{.64} = \$1422.27$

21. $\quad A = Pe^{rt} = 7500(2.718)^{.085(10)} = 7500(2.718)^{.85} = \$17545.80$

25. Use the formula $A = P(1 + \frac{r}{n})^{nt}$ for the first 4 rows. For example, \$1000 at 12% compounded quarterly for 20 years yields

$$A = 1000(1 + \frac{.12}{4})^{4(20)} = 1000(1.03)^{80} = \$10641.$$

Use the formula $A = Pe^{rt}$ for the last row. For example, \$1000 at 12% compounded continuously for 20 years yields

$$A = 1000(2.718)^{.12(20)} = 1000(2.718)^{2.4} = \$11020.$$

29. $f(x) = 2e^x$

The points $(-1, .8)$, $(0,2)$, and $(1, 5.4)$ along with the knowledge of the general shape of an exponential curve should allow you to sketch this curve.

33. $Q(t) = 1000e^{.4t} = 1000(2.718)^{.4(2)} = 1000(2.718)^{.8} = 2225$

$Q(t) = 1000e^{.4t} = 1000(2.718)^{.4(3)} = 1000(2.718)^{1.2} = 3320$

$Q(t) = 1000e^{.4t} = 1000(2.718)^{.4(5)} = 1000(2.718)^{2} = 7388$

Problem Set 10.3

Problems 1-20 are done by applying Definition 10.2.

21. Let $x = \log_2 16$. Now we can change to exponential form and solve.

$$2^x = 16$$
$$2^x = 2^4$$
$$x = 4$$

25. Let $x = \log_6 216$. Now change to exponential form and solve.

$$6^x = 216$$
$$6^x = 6^3$$
$$x = 3$$

29. Let $x = \log_{10} 1$. Now change to exponential form and solve.

$$10^x = 1$$
$$10^x = 10^0$$
$$x = 0$$

33. By direct application of Property 10.4,

$$10^{\log_{10} 5} = 5.$$

37. Let $x = \log_2 32$.

$$2^x = 32$$
$$2^x = 2^5$$
$$x = 5$$

Therefore, $\log_5(\log_2 32)$ becomes $\log_5 5$. Now let $y = \log_5 5$ and switch to exponential form.

$$5^y = 5$$
$$5^y = 5^1$$
$$y = 1$$

Thus, $\log_5(\log_2 32) = 1$.

41. $\log_7 x = 2$

$$7^2 = x$$
$$49 = x$$

The solution set is $\{49\}$.

45. $\log_9 x = \dfrac{3}{2}$

$$9^{\frac{3}{2}} = x$$
$$(\sqrt{9})^3 = x$$
$$3^3 = x$$
$$27 = x$$

The solution set is $\{27\}$.

49. $\log_x 2 = \dfrac{1}{2}$

$$x^{\frac{1}{2}} = 2$$
$$\sqrt{x} = 2$$
$$x = 4$$

The solution set is $\{4\}$.

53. $\log_{10} 49 = \log_{10} 7^2 = 2 \log_{10} 7$
$$= 2(.8451)$$
$$= 1.6902$$

57. $\log_{10} 32 = \log_{10} 2^5 = 5 \log_{10} 2$
$$= 5(.3010)$$
$$= 1.5050$$

61. $\log_{10} 56 = \log_{10}(8 \cdot 7) = \log_{10} 8 + \log_{10} 7$
$$= \log_{10} 2^3 + \log_{10} 7$$
$$= 3 \log_{10} 2 + \log_{10} 7$$
$$= 3(.3010) + .8451 = 1.7481$$

65. $\log_{10} 4900 = \log_{10}(49 \cdot 100) = \log_{10} 49 + \log_{10} 100$
$$= \log_{10} 7^2 + \log_{10} 10^2$$
$$= 2 \log_{10} 7 + 2 = 3.6902$$

69. $\log_b xyz = \log_b x + \log_b y + \log_b z$ by direct application of Property 10.5.

73. $\log_b y^3 z^4 = \log_b y^3 + \log_b z^4$ by Property 10.5 and then by Property 10.7 we can change to $3 \log_b y + 4 \log_b z$.

77. $\log_b \sqrt[3]{x^2 z} = \log_b (x^2 z)^{\frac{1}{3}} = \log_b x^{\frac{2}{3}} z^{\frac{1}{3}}$ by applying earlier properties of exponents. Now we can apply Property 10.5 and Property 10.7.

$$\log_b x^{\frac{2}{3}} z^{\frac{1}{3}} = \log_b x^{\frac{2}{3}} + \log_b z^{\frac{1}{3}} = \frac{2}{3} \log_b x + \frac{1}{3} \log_b z$$

81. $\log_{10} x + \log_{10} 25 = 2$

$$\log_{10} 25x = 2 \qquad \text{Property 10.5}$$

$$10^2 = 25x \qquad \text{Change to exponential form.}$$
$$100 = 25x$$
$$4 = x$$

The solution set is $\{4\}$.

85. $\log_{10}x + \log_{10}(x-21) = 2$

$$\log_{10}x(x-21) = 2 \qquad \text{Property 10.5}$$

$$10^2 = x(x-21) \qquad \text{Change to exponential form.}$$

$$100 = x^2-21x$$

$$0 = x^2-21x-100$$

$$0 = (x-25)(x+4)$$

$$x-25 = 0 \text{ or } x+4 = 0$$

$$x = 25 \text{ or } \quad x = -4$$

Since logarithms of negative numbers are not defined, the -4 solution must be discarded. Thus, the solution set is $\{25\}$.

89. $\log_{10}(2x-1) - \log_{10}(x-2) = 1$

$$\log_{10}\frac{2x-1}{x-2} = 1 \qquad \text{Property 10.6}$$

$$10^1 = \frac{2x-1}{x-2} \qquad \text{Change to exponential form.}$$

$$10x-20 = 2x-1$$

$$8x = 19$$

$$x = \frac{19}{8}$$

The solution set is $\{\frac{19}{8}\}$.

Problem Set 10.4

1. The equation $y = \log_{\frac{1}{2}}x$ can be written in exponential form as $(\frac{1}{2})^y = x$.
Now the points $(1,0),(\frac{1}{2},1),(\frac{1}{4},2),(2,-1)$, and $(4,-2)$ can be used to help sketch the curve.

5. (a) The graph of $f(x) = 1 + \log_{10}x$ is the graph of $f(x) = \log_{10}x$ shifted up one unit. The points $(1,1),(10,2)$, and $(.1,0)$ should help with the sketch.

17. $\log 4.94 = .6937$ by reading directly from the table.

21. $\log 409 = \log(4.09 \cdot 10^2)$

$$= \log 4.09 + \log 10^2$$

$$= \log 4.09 + 2 \log 10$$

$$= .6117 + 2$$

$$= 2.6117$$

25. $\log .00177 = \log(1.77 \cdot 10^{-3})$

$$= \log 1.77 + \log 10^{-3}$$

$$= \log 1.77 + (-3) \log 10$$

$$= .2480 + (-3)$$

41. $\text{antilog } 1.4829 = \text{antilog}(.4829 + 1)$

$$= (3.04)(10)^1$$

$$= 30.4$$

45. antilog 5.8062 = antilog (.8062 + 5)

$$= (6.40)(10)^5$$

$$= 640{,}000$$

49. antilog (-3 + .8639) = $(10^{-3})(7.31)$

$$= .00731$$

Problem Set 10.5

13. ln 7.2 = 1.9741 by reading directly from the table.

17. $\ln 740 = \ln (7.4 \cdot 10^2)$

$$= \ln 7.4 + \ln 10^2$$

$$= \ln 7.4 + 2\ln 10$$

$$= 2.0015 + 2(2.3026)$$

$$= 6.6067$$

21. $\ln .0082 = \ln(8.2 \cdot 10^{-3})$

$$= \ln 8.2 + \ln 10^{-3}$$

$$= \ln 8.2 + (-3) \ln 10$$

$$= 2.1041 - 6.9078$$

$$= -4.8037$$

25.

$$4^x = 21$$

$$\ln 4^x = \ln 21$$

$$x \ln 4 = \ln 21$$

$$x = \frac{\ln 21}{\ln 4} = 2.20 \text{ to the nearest hundredth}$$

The solution set is {2.20}.

29.

$$5^{3x+1} = 9$$

$$\ln 5^{3x+1} = \ln 9$$

$$(3x+1)\ln 5 = \ln 9$$

$$3x \ln 5 + \ln 5 = \ln 9$$

$$3x \ln 5 = \ln 9 - \ln 5$$

$$x = \frac{\ln 9 - \ln 5}{3 \ln 5} = .12 \text{ to the nearest hundredth}$$

The solution set is {.12}.

33.

$$e^{x-2} = 13.1$$

$$\ln e^{x-2} = \ln 13.1$$

$$(x-2)\ln e = \ln 13.1$$

$$x-2 = \ln 13.1 \qquad (\ln e = 1)$$

$$x = \ln 13.1 + 2$$

$$x = 2.57 + 2 = 4.57 \quad \text{to the nearest hundredth}$$

The solution set is {4.57}.

37. Let x = $\log_2 23$ which can be written in exponential form as $2^x = 23$.

$$2^x = 23$$
$$\ln 2^x = \ln 23$$
$$x \ln 2 = \ln 23$$
$$x = \frac{\ln 23}{\ln 2} = 4.524$$

41. Let x = $\log_7 421$ which can be written in exponential form as $7^x = 421$.

$$7^x = 421$$
$$\ln 7^x = \ln 421$$
$$x \ln 7 = \ln 421$$
$$x = \frac{\ln 421}{\ln 7} = 3.105$$

45. Let x = $\log_3 720$ which can be written in exponential form as $3^x = 720$.

$$3^x = 720$$
$$\ln 3^x = \ln 720$$
$$x \ln 3 = \ln 720$$
$$x = \frac{\ln 720}{\ln 3} = 5.989$$

49. Use the formula $A = Pe^{rt}$.

$$4000 = 2000e^{.13t}$$
$$2 = e^{.13t}$$
$$\ln 2 = \ln e^{.13t}$$
$$\ln 2 = .13t \ln e$$
$$\ln 2 = .13t \qquad (\ln e = 1)$$
$$\frac{\ln 2}{.13} = t$$
$$5.3 = t$$

53. Use the formula $Q = Q_0 e^{.34t}$.

$$4000 = 400e^{.34t}$$
$$10 = e^{.34t}$$
$$\ln 10 = \ln e^{.34t}$$
$$\ln 10 = .34t(\ln e)$$
$$\ln 10 = .34t \qquad (\ln e = 1)$$
$$\frac{\ln 10}{.34} = t$$
$$6.8 = t$$

Chapter 11

Problem Set 11.1

1. $a_n = 3n-4$

$a_1 = 3(1)-4 = -1, \quad a_2 = 3(2)-4 = 2, \quad a_3 = 3(3)-4 = 5,$

$a_4 = 3(4)-4 = 8, \quad a_5 = 3(5)-4 = 11$

5. $a_n = n^2-2$

$a_1 = 1^2-2 = -1, \quad a_2 = 2^2-2 = 2, \quad a_3 = 3^2-2 = 7$

$a_4 = 4^2-2 = 14, \quad a_5 = 5^2-2 = 23$

9. $a_n = 2n^2-3$

$a_1 = 2(1)^2-3 = -1, \quad a_2 = 2(2)^2-3 = 5, \quad a_3 = 2(3)^2-3 = 15,$

$a_4 = 2(4)^2-3 = 29, \quad a_5 = 2(5)^2-3 = 47$

13. $a_n = -2(3)^{n-2}$

$a_1 = -2(3)^{1-2} = -2(3)^{-1} = -2\left(\frac{1}{3}\right) = -\frac{2}{3}$

$a_2 = -2(3)^{2-2} = -2(3)^0 = -2(1) = -2$

$a_3 = -2(3)^{3-2} = -2(3)^1 = -6$

$a_4 = -2(3)^{4-2} = -2(3)^2 = -18$

$a_5 = -2(3)^{5-2} = -2(3)^3 = -54$

17. $a_n = (-2)^{n-2}$

$a_7 = (-2)^{7-2} = (-2)^5 = -32$

$a_8 = (-2)^{8-2} = (-2)^6 = 64$

21. Substitute -2 for a_1 and 4 for d in the formula $a_n = a_1+(n-1)d$.

$a_n = -2+(n-1)4$

$= -2+4n-4$

$= 4n-6$

25. Substitute -7 for a_1 and -3 for d in the formula $a_n = a_1+(n-1)d$.

$a_n = -7+(n-1)(-3)$

$= -7-3n+3$

$= -3n-4$

29. Use the formula $a_n = a_1 + (n-1)d$.

$$a_{10} = 7 + 9(3) = 34$$

33. Use the formula $a_n = a_1 + (n-1)d$.

$$a_{75} = -7 + (74)(-2) = -7 - 148 = -155$$

37. Substitute 157 for a_n, 10 for a_1, and 3 for d in the formula $a_n = a_1 + (n-1)d$.

$$157 = 10 + (n-1)3$$
$$157 = 10 + 3n - 3$$
$$157 = 7 + 3n$$
$$150 = 3n$$
$$50 = n$$

41. $a_6 = 24 = a_1 + 5d$ and $a_{10} = 44 = a_1 + 9d$

Solving the system $\begin{pmatrix} a_1 + 5d = 24 \\ a_1 + 9d = 44 \end{pmatrix}$ produces $a_1 = -1$ and $d = 5$. Thus,

the first term is -1.

45. Substitute 5.02 for a_n, .97 for a_1, and .03 for d in $a_n = a_1 + (n-1)d$.

$$5.02 = .97 + (n-1).03$$
$$502 = 97 + 3n - 3$$
$$408 = 3n$$
$$136 = n$$

49. The sequence 900,930,960,... represents the monthly salary at 6-month intervals. The 10th term of this sequence will represent your monthly salary during the last 6-month period of the 5 year cycle.

$$a_{10} = 900 + 9(30) = \$1170$$

Problem Set 11.2

1. $2+4+6+8+...$

$$a_{50} = 2 + 49(2) = 100$$

$$S_{50} = \frac{50}{2}(2+100) = 25(102) = 2550$$

5. $(-1)+(-3)+(-5)+...$

$$a_{65} = -1 + 64(-2) = -129$$

$$S_{65} = \frac{65}{2}(-1+(-129)) = \frac{65}{2}(-130) = -4225$$

9. $7+10+13+16+...$

$$a_{75} = 7 + 74(3) = 229$$

$$S_{75} = \frac{75}{2}(7+229) = \frac{75}{2}(236) = 8850$$

13. We can use $a_n = a_1+(n-1)d$ to find the number of terms.

$$173 = -4+(n-1)3$$
$$173 = -4+3n-3$$
$$180 = 3n$$
$$60 = n$$

Now we can use the sum formula.

$$S_{60} = \frac{60}{2}(-4+173) = 30(169) = 5070$$

17. We can use $a_n = 3n-1$ to find the 1st and 50th terms.

$$a_1 = 3(1)-1 = 2 \text{ and } a_{50} = 3(50)-1 = 149$$

Now we can use the sum formula.

$$S_{50} = \frac{50}{2}(2+149) = 25(151) = 3775$$

21. We can use $a_n = -4n-1$ to find the 1st and 65th terms.

$$a_1 = -4(1)-1 = -5 \text{ and } a_{65} = -4(65)-1 = -261$$

Now we can use the sum formula.

$$S_{65} = \frac{65}{2}(-5+(-261)) = \frac{65}{2}(-266) = -8645$$

25. $15+17+19+...+397$

We can use $a_n = a_1+(n-1)d$ to find the number of terms.

$$397 = 15+2(n-1)$$
$$397 = 15+2n-2$$
$$384 = 2n$$
$$192 = n$$

Now we can use the sum formula.

$$S_{192} = \frac{192}{2}(15+397) = 39552$$

29. The series $1+3+5+...$ represents the money (in cents) to be taken in by the raffle.

We can use $a_n = a_1+(n-1)d$ to find the 1000th term.

$$a_{1000} = 1+(999)2 = 1999$$

Now we can use the sum formula.

$$S_{1000} = \frac{1000}{2}(1+1999) = 1,000,000 \text{ cents}$$

Thus, in dollars we have $10,000.

33. The series $25+23+21+...+1$ represents the pile of cans.

$$S_{13} = \frac{13}{2}(25+1) = \frac{13}{2}(26) = 169$$

<u>Problem Set 11.3</u>

1. Substitute 1 for a_1 and 3 for r in the formula $a_n = a_1 r^{n-1}$.

$$a_n = 1(3)^{n-1} = 3^{n-1}$$

5. Substitute 1 for a_1 and $\frac{1}{3}$ for r in the formula $a_n = a_1 r^{n-1}$.

$$a_n = 1\left(\frac{1}{3}\right)^{n-1} = \frac{1}{3^{n-1}}$$

9. Substitute 9 for a_1 and $\frac{2}{3}$ for r in the formula $a_n = a_1 r^{n-1}$.

$$a_n = 9\left(\frac{2}{3}\right)^{n-1} = \frac{(9)(2)^{n-1}}{3^{n-1}} = \frac{3^2(2)^{n-1}}{3^{n-1}} = (3^{3-n})(2)^{n-1}$$

13. Substitute $\frac{1}{9}$ for a_1, 3 for r, and 12 for n in the formula $a_n = a_1 r^{n-1}$.

$$a_{12} = \frac{1}{9}(3)^{11} = 19{,}683$$

17. Substitute -1 for a, $\frac{3}{2}$ for r, and 9 for n in the formula $a_n = a_1 r^{n-1}$.

$$a_9 = -1\left(\frac{3}{2}\right)^8 = -\frac{6561}{256}$$

21. Substitute -2 for a_1, -3 for r, and 9 for n in the sum formula.

$$S_n = \frac{a_1 r^n - a_1}{r-1} = \frac{a_1(r^n-1)}{r-1}$$

$$S_9 = \frac{-2((-3)^9-1)}{-3-1} = \frac{-2(-19684)}{-4} = -9842$$

25. We can use $a_n = 2^{n-1}$ to find the first term.

$$a_1 = 2^{1-1} = 2^0 = 1$$

Now we can use the sum formula.

$$S_9 = \frac{1(2^9-1)}{2-1} = 511$$

29. We can use $a_n = (-2)^n$ to find the first term.

$$a_1 = (-2)^1 = -2$$

Now we can use the sum formula.

$$S_{12} = \frac{-2((-2)^{12}-1)}{-2-1} = \frac{(-2)(4095)}{-3} = 2730$$

33. $1 + \dfrac{1}{2} + \dfrac{1}{4} + \ldots + \dfrac{1}{1024}$

Solution A

The number of terms can be found using $a_n = a_1 r^{n-1}$.

$$\frac{1}{1024} = 1\left(\frac{1}{2}\right)^{n-1}$$

$$\left(\frac{1}{2}\right)^{10} = \left(\frac{1}{2}\right)^{n-1}$$

$$n-1 = 10$$

$$n = 11$$

Now we can use the sum formula.

$$S_{11} = \frac{1\left(\left(\frac{1}{2}\right)^{11} - 1\right)}{\frac{1}{2} - 1} = \frac{\frac{1}{2048} - 1}{-\frac{1}{2}} = \frac{-\frac{2047}{2048}}{-\frac{1}{2}} = \frac{2047}{1024} = 1\frac{1023}{1024}$$

Solution B

We can also do this type of problem by using the approach illustrated in Example 3 of the text.

$$S = 1 + \frac{1}{2} + \frac{1}{4} + \ldots + \frac{1}{1024} \qquad (1)$$

Multiply both sides by the common ratio, $\dfrac{1}{2}$.

$$\frac{1}{2}S = \frac{1}{2} + \frac{1}{4} + \ldots + \frac{1}{1024} + \frac{1}{2048} \qquad (2)$$

Subtract equation (2) from equation (1).

$$\frac{1}{2}S = 1 - \frac{1}{2048}$$

$$\frac{1}{2}S = \frac{2047}{2048}$$

$$S = \left(\frac{2047}{2048}\right)(2) = \frac{2047}{1024} = 1\frac{1023}{1024}$$

37. The formula $a_n = a_1 r^{n-1}$ can be used to generate two equations.

$$a_2 = a_1 r^1 = \frac{1}{6}$$

$$a_5 = a_1 r^4 = \frac{1}{48}$$

$$\frac{a_1 r^4}{a_1 r^1} = \frac{\frac{1}{48}}{\frac{1}{6}}$$

$$r^3 = \frac{1}{8}$$

$$r = \frac{1}{2}$$

41. The sequence 8000,4000,2000,... represents how much water remains after the 1st day, 2nd day, and so on. Thus, we want to find the 7th term of this sequence.

$$a_7 = 8000\left(\frac{1}{2}\right)^6 = 8000\left(\frac{1}{64}\right) = 125$$

Therefore, 125 liters remain after 7 days.

45. Sometimes a very simple diagram helps with the analysis of a problem. Let's draw a diagram here to represent the "bouncing ball."

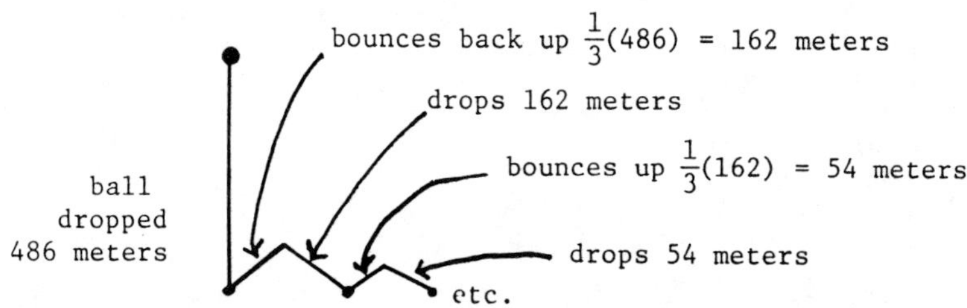

Let's set up a series so that each term represents a "roundtrip" up and down. Then we can add 486 meters that represents the first drop.

324+108+36+...

Let's find the sum of the first 6 terms of this series.

$$S_6 = \frac{324\left(\left(\frac{1}{3}\right)^6 - 1\right)}{\frac{1}{3} - 1} = \frac{324\left(\frac{1}{729} - 1\right)}{-\frac{2}{3}}$$

$$= -\frac{3}{2}(324)\left(-\frac{728}{729}\right)$$

$$= 485.\overline{3}$$

Therefore, the total distance is $485.\overline{3} + 486 = 971.\overline{3}$ meters.

Problem Set 11.4

1. $1 + \frac{3}{4} + \frac{9}{16} + \frac{27}{64} + \ldots$

$$S_\infty = \frac{a_1}{1-r} = \frac{1}{1 - \frac{3}{4}} = \frac{1}{\frac{1}{4}} = 4$$

5. $\frac{2}{3} + \frac{4}{9} + \frac{8}{27} + \frac{16}{81} + \ldots$

$$S_\infty = \frac{a_1}{1-r} = \frac{\frac{2}{3}}{1 - \frac{2}{3}} = \frac{\frac{2}{3}}{\frac{1}{3}} = 2$$

9. $6 + 2 + \frac{2}{3} + \frac{2}{9} + \ldots$

$$S_\infty = \frac{a_1}{1-r} = \frac{6}{1 - \frac{1}{3}} = \frac{6}{\frac{2}{3}} = 9$$

13. $1 + \left(-\frac{3}{4}\right) + \frac{9}{16} + \left(-\frac{27}{64}\right) + \ldots$

$$S_\infty = \frac{a_1}{1-r} = \frac{1}{1 - \left(-\frac{3}{4}\right)}$$

$$= \frac{1}{1 + \frac{3}{4}} = \frac{1}{\frac{7}{4}} = \frac{4}{7}$$

17. Since $r = \frac{3}{2}$, this series has no sum.

21. The repeating decimal $.\overline{4}$ can be written as an infinite geometric series

$$.4 + .04 + .004 + \ldots$$

with $a_1 = .4$ and $r = .1$.

$$S_\infty = \frac{a_1}{1-r} = \frac{.4}{1 - .1} = \frac{.4}{.9} = \frac{4}{9}$$

Therefore, $.\overline{4} = \frac{4}{9}$.

25. The repeating decimal $.\overline{45}$ can be written as an infinite geometric series

$$.45 + .0045 + .000045 + \ldots$$

with $a_1 = .45$ and $r = .01$.

$$S_\infty = \frac{a_1}{1-r} = \frac{.45}{1 - .01} = \frac{.45}{.99} = \frac{45}{99} = \frac{5}{11}$$

Therefore, $.\overline{45} = \frac{5}{11}$.

29. The repeating decimal $.4\overline{6}$ can be written as

$$[.4] + [.06 + .006 + .0006 + \ldots]$$

where $.06 + .006 + .0006 + \ldots$ is an infinite geometric series with $a_1 = .06$ and $r = .1$.

$$S_\infty = \frac{a_1}{1-r} = \frac{.06}{1 - .1} = \frac{.06}{.9} = \frac{6}{90} = \frac{1}{15}$$

Therefore, $.4\overline{6} = .4 + \frac{1}{15} = \frac{4}{10} + \frac{1}{15} = \frac{2}{5} + \frac{1}{15} = \frac{7}{15}$.

33. The repeating decimal $.4\overline{27}$ can be written as

$$[.4] + [.027 + .00027 + .0000027 + \ldots]$$

where $.027 + .00027 + .0000027 + \ldots$ is any infinite geometric series with $a_1 = .027$ and $r = .01$.

$$S = \frac{a_1}{1-r} = \frac{.027}{1 - .01} = \frac{.027}{.99} = \frac{27}{990} = \frac{3}{110}$$

Therefore, $.4\overline{27} = .4 + \frac{3}{110}$

$$= \frac{4}{10} + \frac{3}{110}$$

$$= \frac{47}{110}$$

<u>Problem Set 11.5</u>

For Problems 1-6 you are to use Pascal's triangle to determine the coefficients.

1. $(x+y)^8 = x^8+8x^7y+28x^6y^2+56x^5y^3+70x^4y^4+56x^3y^5+28x^2y^6+8xy^7+y^8$

5. $(x-y)^5 = x^5-5x^4y+10x^3y^2-10x^2y^3+5xy^4-y^5$

9. $(2x+y)^6 = (2x)^6+6(2x)^5(y) +\dfrac{6\cdot5}{2!}(2x)^4(y)^2$

$$+ \dfrac{6\cdot5\cdot4}{3!}(2x)^3(y)^3 + \dfrac{6\cdot5\cdot4\cdot3}{4!}(2x)^2(y)^4$$

$$+ \dfrac{6\cdot5\cdot4\cdot3\cdot2}{5!}(2x)(y)^5 +y^6$$

$$= 64x^6+192x^5y+240x^4y^2+160x^3y^3+60x^2y^4+12xy^5+y^6$$

13. $(3a-2b)^5 = (3a)^5+5(3a)^4(-2b) +\dfrac{5\cdot4}{2!}(3a)^3(-2b)^2$

$$+\dfrac{5\cdot4\cdot3}{3!}(3a)^2(-2b)^3 +\dfrac{5\cdot4\cdot3\cdot2}{4!}(3a)(-2b)^4 + (-2b)^5$$

$$= 243a^5-810a^4b+1080a^3b^2-720a^2b^3+240ab^4-32b^5$$

17. $(x+2)^7 = x^7 + 7x^6(2) +\dfrac{7\cdot6}{2!}x^5(2)^2 + \dfrac{7\cdot6\cdot6}{3!}x^4(2)^3$

$$+ \dfrac{7\cdot6\cdot5\cdot4}{4!}x^3(2)^4 + \dfrac{7\cdot6\cdot5\cdot4\cdot3}{5!}x^2(2)^5 + \dfrac{7\cdot6\cdot5\cdot4\cdot3\cdot2}{6!}x(2)^6+ (2)^7$$

$$= x^7+14x^6+84x^5+280x^4+560x^3+672x^2+448x+128$$

21. The first four terms of $(x+y)^{15}$ are

$$x^{15}+15x^{14}y +\dfrac{15\cdot14}{2!}x^{13}y^2+ \dfrac{15\cdot14\cdot13}{3!}x^{12}y^3$$

which simplifies to

$$x^{15}+15x^{14}y+105x^{13}y^2+455x^{12}y^3 .$$

25. The 7th term of $(x+y)^{11}$ contains y^6 and therefore also contains x^5. The coefficient is

$$\dfrac{11\cdot10\cdot9\cdot8\cdot7\cdot6}{6!} = 462 .$$

Therefore, the 7th term is $462x^5y^6$.

29. The 3rd term of $(2x-5y)^5$ contains $(-5y)^2$ and $(2x)^3$. The coefficient is

$$\dfrac{5\cdot4}{2!} = \dfrac{5\cdot4}{2} = 10 .$$

Therefore, the 3rd term is $2000x^3y^2$.

Keto Diet for Beginners:

TOP 51 Amazing and Simple Recipes in One Ketogenic Cookbook,

Any Recipes on Your Choice for Any Meal Time

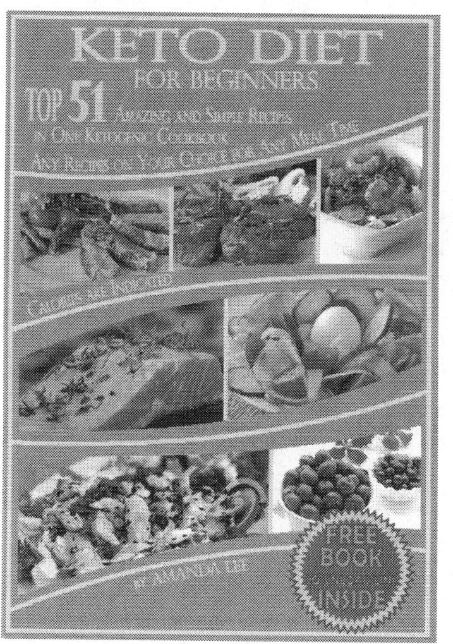

Get Your Free Bonus

I wanted to show my appreciation that you support my work so I've put together a bonus for you.

Keto Diet for Beginners:

Ketogenic Smoothie and Dessert Recipes

Just visit the link or scan QR-code to download it now:

https://wondergoodsfactory.com/landing-pages/amanda-lee-free-bonus-download/

Thanks!

Amanda Lee

Table of Contents

Introduction

Do you suffer from obesity? The rising incidence of obesity is taking its toll on the health of a large population segment. While we do believe that people of all sizes are beautiful, you must pay heed to a growing waistline because being overweight is never healthy.

There are countless methods to lose weight, but traditional crash diets and starving yourself are definitely the wrong routes to pursue. This is why we want to introduce you to the ketogenic diet. It's one of the smarter dieting methods wherein you still lower your caloric intake, but do so intelligently in order to provide your body with vital nutrients and avoid complications.

A ketogenic diet is a balanced form of dieting that's-become increasingly popular due to the positive benefits it offers. It's a healthy way of shedding extra pounds because it doesn't deplete muscle, but simply works on the extra unwanted layers of fat and discards them.

In this book we're going to provide you comprehensive details regarding what this diet entails and how you can stick to it, all while enjoying your meals and shedding the extra pounds that seem to have piled on. Does it sound too good to be true? Let's get to facts and prove the benefits to you.

Chapter 1: What Is A Ketogenic Diet?

A ketogenic diet, also colloquially known as keto, is one where you decrease your daily intake of carbohydrates in order to burn body fat. This is far different from a crash diet because you don't skip meals or make them smaller.

Keto mainly involves minimizing the consumption of carbohydrates by regulating the kind of food you eat. Doing this forces your body to enter the state of ketosis. This state is where the ketogenic diet derives its name, and leads us to explain what ketosis actually is.

Ketosis – The Term Explained

Ketosis is mainly a state in which your body is forced to break fat molecules down into smaller molecules, known as ketones. These ketones are then used by the body to generate energy for carrying out different activities. Ketosis is achieved by decreasing carbohydrate intake.

The usual state your body is in is known as glycolysis.While in glycolysis, carbohydrates (carbs) are broken down into smaller and simpler substances to produce energy. As long as carbs are available, the body makes little use of stored fat molecules. However, if you reduce carb intake significantly, the body turns to stored fat as an energy source, thereby entering ketosis.

Hence, the ketogenic diet's principle element consists of pursuing a diet strictly low in carbohydrates. Apart from helping you achieve weight loss, you can also experience various other health benefits.

Keto Flu

This said, it is important to note that, like all forms of dieting, you will likely experience some form of initial discomfort.

At the outset, your body may take some time to adjust to altered eating patterns. You may experience some or all of the below symptoms.

- Headaches
- Lethargy
- Sluggishness
- Gastrointestinal issues

This phase is known as the keto flu. There is no reason to panic, because it tends to subside in a couple of weeks after your body adapts to your new eating habits. If you initiate a balanced electrolyte intake program, this problem often subsides even more quickly.

One of the key reasons people tend to opt for keto is the diminished loss of muscle common with other dieting methods. So, if you are looking for a healthy way to shed extra pounds without forcing your body into a state of extreme weakness, a ketogenic diet might be for you.

Chapter 2: Aspects of Keto

Potential Pitfalls

If you've decided to attempt keto, you should be well acquainted with certain aspects. Here are two caveats you should keep in mind.

Do not combine keto with other dieting methods. For example: crash dieting will result in loss of muscle and nutrient deprivation, making both your body physically weak and stressing your immune system, leaving you more susceptible to illness. While this additional caloric restriction in conjunction with keto might result in rapid fat loss, the negative effects will increase commensurately, putting your health at risk.

• The initial week or two might be somewhat trying for your body. Properly attend to yourself by consuming an adequate amount of water and nutrient rich vegetables.

Useful tips

It can be too hard to adhere the diet strictly in first few weeks. The temptation to eat something sweet, tasty and forbidden is all around you and it's difficult to stand against. However, if you want to achieve the desired results, it's extremely necessary to show all your will and be strict with yourself. This is the only way to succeed in your goal. Methods of self-discipline development may become a substantial help in achieving the desired results. There are many works which are devoted to this subject, but I'd like to recommend you "Daily Self-Discipline" book by Emily Clemons. This is a really great book that will strengthen your willpower and teach you how to get rid of bad habits just in a few couple weeks and to achieve your goals.

And moreover, the techniques and tips that are presented in Emily's book are applicable not only for the diet but almost for all aspects of life. Just click this link or scan QR-code for more information about the contents of this book.

Go to the "Daily Self-Discipline" by Emily Clemons

Incentives

A ketogenic diet aids in healthy loss of weight without excessive muscle wasting. Your body will retain the capacity to carry out normal daily activities. With the addition of higher protein consumption and regular exercise, it's even possible to gain lean muscle tissue while burning fat quicker. So, if you're a fitness buff looking for ways to stay consistently healthy and fit, you should definitely delve deeper into the dynamics of keto.

Additionally, scientific research has found that people following a ketogenic diet show improvements with regard to maintaining proper blood sugar levels. Thus, patients suffering from diabetes are also potential candidates for keto. Those suffering from high blood pressure can see major reductions during diet initiation, while facilitating stability and regulation long term. Others with heart disease will find that keto tends to curb the level of triglycerides in the body while showing a decrease in the level of LDL cholesterol and even blood glucose. HDL (the 'good') cholesterol tends to increase.

Now, while this next point doesn't currently have ample conclusive evidence, research has indicated that a ketogenic diet is known to starve cancer cells, aiding in curtailing the growth of tumours. Nutrient dense cancer-fighting foods commonly part of keto only serve to bolster therapeutic claims. As you can see, the potential benefits this diet could impart are extensive.

Nutrients to incorporate in your diet

Before going into the details of recipes for preparing meals consistent with a ketogenic diet, we'll discuss some of the ingredients frequently used. Knowing this will give you a snapshot of food items best utilized or avoided.

Seafood

If you're a seafood lover, you have every reason to smile. Seafood, mainly fish and shellfish, are rich sources of protein and omega 3 fatty acids advocated in keto. But, the carbohydrate content in shellfish tends to vary somewhat. Gauge the potential carb intake by researching the particular species before purchase.

Ideally, two servings of seafood every week are recommended. Salmon, mackerel, and sardines are top choices.

Cheese

If you wondered if you read that heading correctly, rest assured you did. Cheese is actually very low in carb content and high in fat. It contains conjugated linoleum acid (CLA), a type of fat comprehensively shown to have several different anti-obesity mechanisms resulting in body fat reduction and improved overall body composition, making it one of the best foods for keto.

Eggs

Eggs are definitely on the keto chart. A large egg contains less than 1 gram of carbohydrate. Their consumption is known to trigger specific hormones that give you a feeling your appetite has been satiated, which could help you cut superfluous calorie intake. Eggs also aid in stabilizing blood sugar levels, definitely making them a good option.

Low Carb Vegetables

There are a lot of non-starchy vegetables known to be low in both calories and carbs while being extremely nutrient dense. Cruciferous vegetables like broccoli, cauliflower, kale are very good choices.

Avoid starchy vegetables such as potatoes, corn, yams, pumpkin, squash, and zucchini. We know potatoes are a staple part of many diets, but even a small serving could fulfill your carb intake for he day.

Animal Proteins

Animal proteins like meat and fish have an extremely small amount of carbs. They come in handy o sate hunger pangs and you should consume moderate amounts. Further, organ meats like liver, heart, and bone marrow are also low carb, with greater mineral content, making them good candidates. Lamb, goat, venison and even grass fed beef seem to be good options for ketogenic diet followers.

These are some of the food groups you need to stick with when implementing a ketogenic diet. They'll help you derive the greatest benefits from this form of regimen.

Chapter 3: Recipes. Ketogenic Breakfast

Here, are 51 great recipes to ensure you'll be able to enjoy food, despite dieting. We'll be sharing recipes for breakfast, snacks, lunch, and dinner so you can keep munching a bit whenever you want.

Let's start with some of the most delectable breakfast recipes that will help you kick start your day the right way.

1. Keto Cereal

This keto cereal is a healthy choice for everyone who is looking to shed extra pounds without comprising on taste.

Ingredients

- ½ cup of shredded coconut (40 g)
- 2 cups of almond milk (480g)
- 1/3 cup of crushed walnut piece (39g)
- 1/3 cup of toasted flaxseeds (55g)
- 3 to 4 tsp of butter (17g)
- Erythritol (8g)
- Salt (4g)

Instructions

- Melt the butter on medium heat.
- Add the nuts and salt to the melted butter and stir for a couple of minutes.
- Add shredded coconut and keep mixing. Make sure the bottom doesn't start to burn.
- To this mixture, add the sweetener of your choice. Ideally, it shouldn't be more than 1 tbsp.
- Now, quickly add your milk.
- Stir and turn off the heat.

Note: Do not add too many nuts as it might defeat the purpose of following a ketogenic diet.

Servings quantity: 2	Weight:
Energy (calories): Total = 889.00 kcal	Total = 643.00 g Per one serving = 321.50 g
Per one serving = 444.50 kcal	**Total carbohydrate:** Total = 31.82 g Per one serving = 15.91 g
Calorie breakdown: Protein: 8% / 73.00 kcal Fat: 78% / 691.00 kcal Carbohydrates: 13% / 119.00 kcal	Protein: Total = 20.51 g / p.s. = 10.26 g
Carbohydrates mass fraction: 4.95%	Fat: Total = 81.39 g / p.s. = 40.70 g

2. Keto Bagel

Bagels are always a satisfying choice. Far from your normal bagel, this recipe will definitely help you with a healthy and tasty start.

Ingredients

- ½ cup hemp hearts (80g)
- ¼ cup psyllium fibre (13g)
- 6 egg whites, organic (198g)
- 1 cup coconut flour (114g)
- ½ cup sesame seeds (75g)
- ½ cup pumpkin seeds (32g)
- 1 tbsp baking powder (4g)
- 1 tsp Celtic sea salt (6g)

Instructions

- Preheat the oven to 350 degrees.
- Take a large bowl and mix all the ingredients in it.
- Blend the egg whites in a blender until you get a foamy mixture.
- Pour the egg whites into the well-churned dry ingredients and mix until smooth.
- Add a cup of boiling water and keep stirring until a smooth dough forms.
- Now place parchment paper on a cookie sheet.
- Divide the dough into 6 balls of roughly equal size.
- With your finger, make a hole in each ball then press the dough onto the cookie sheet, giving it the shape of a bagel.
- Sprinkle a bit of sesame seeds on top.
- Bake them for 55 minutes at 350 degrees.

Servings quantity: 6 bagels	Weight:
Energy (calories): Total = 1736.00 kcal	Total = 559.00 g Per one serving = 93.17 g
Per one serving = 289.33 kcal	**Total carbohydrate:**
Calorie breakdown:	Total = 35.04 g
Protein: 16% / 271.00 kcal Fat: 74% / 1282.00 kcal	Per one serving = 5.84 g
Carbohydrates: 11% / 183.00 kcal	Protein: Total = 72.51 g / p.s. = 12.09 g
Carbohydrates mass fraction: 6.27%	Fat: Total = 153.10 g / p.s. = 25.52 g

3. Eggs and Vegetables

This is a fitting start! It has just the right amount of calories to provide much needed daily energy.

Ingredients

- 80g carrots
- 3 eggs (132g)
- 100g cauliflower
- 100g spinach
- 1tbsp coconut oil (14g)
- 100g broccoli
- 100g green beans
- spices (8g)

Instructions

- Add just enough coconut oil to coat the frying pan bottom.
- Heat gently.
- Add vegetables. If using a frozen mix, thaw on low heat for a few minutes,
- Increase heat to medium.
- Add 3 eggs.
- Add various spices to taste.
- Stir fry until ready to serve.

Servings quantity: 2	Weight:
Energy (calories): Total = 470.00 kcal	Total = 634.00 g Per one serving = 317.00 g
Per one serving = 235.00 kcal	**Total carbohydrate:**
Calorie breakdown: Protein: 21% / 101.00 kcal	Total = 31.21 g Per one serving = 15.61 g
Fat: 53% / 251.00 kcal	
Carbohydrates: 25% / 118.00 kcal	Protein: Total = 27.75 g / p.s. = 13.88 g
Carbohydrates mass fraction: 4.92%	Fat: Total = 28.59 g / p.s. = 14.30 g

4. Low Carb Ham & Cheese Stuffed Waffles

If you thought waffles were just dessert for breakfast, it's time to reconsider.

Ingredients

- 7 tbsp of almond milk (105g)
- 2 eggs (88g)
- ¾ cup of almond flour (71g)
- 2 ½ tbsp of coconut flour (15g)
- ½ tsp of apple cider vinegar (3g)
- 2 tsp of corn free baking powder (9g)
- ½ tsp of vanilla extract (2g)
- 4 slices of deli ham (92g)
- 1 tbsp of coconut oil (14g)
- 2 tsp of erythritol (8g)
- 4 slices of cheddar cheese (112g)

Instructions

- Preheat the waffle iron to medium high.
- In large mixing bowl, stir almond milk and apple cider vinegar together.
- Add eggs, olive oil, coconut, and vanilla extract and mix thoroughly.
- In a different mixing bowl, add coconut flour, almond flour, baking powder and 2 tsp sweetener. Whisk together.
- Now, add dry flour to the egg mixture and whisk thoroughly.
- Pour approximately ¼ of batter into the waffle iron, making sure it's uniformly spread.
- On top of the batter, place 2 slices of ham, then 2 slices of cheese.
- Add a little more batter.
- Close the iron and cook for 3 to 5 minutes.

Servings quantity: 2	Weight:
Energy (calories): Total = 1368.00 kcal	Total = 519.00 g Per one serving = 259.50 g
Per one serving = 684.00 kcal	**Total carbohydrate:**
Calorie breakdown:	Total = 26.61 g
Protein: 20% / 278.00 kcal	Per one serving = 13.31 g
Fat: 70% / 953.00 kcal	
Carbohydrates: 7% / 100.94 kcal	Protein: Total = 70.54 g / p.s. = 35.27 g
Carbohydrates mass fraction: 5.13%	Fat: Total = 109.57 g / p.s. = 54.79 g

5. Green Low Carb Breakfast Smoothie

For those who love smoothies, this low carb version will definitely help you stick to your keto diet plan with something delicious to sip on.

Ingredients

- 1 oz of spinach (28g)
- 50 g of celery
- 1 ½ cups of almond milk (360g)
- 50 g of avocado
- 50 g of cucumber
- 1 tbsp coconut oil (14g)
- 1 scoop of protein powder (30 g)
- 10 drops of liquid stevia (10g)
- ½ tsp of chia seeds (3g)

Instructions

- Add almond milk and spinach to blender.
- Blend briefly.
- Add the rest of the ingredients to the slightly blended mixture and blend thoroughly.
- Pour mixture in glass and sprinkle chia seeds on top.

Servings quantity: 2	Weight:
Energy (calories): Total = 410.00 kcal	Total = 595.00 g Per one serving = 297.50 g
Per one serving = 205.00 kcal	**Total carbohydrate:**
Calorie breakdown:	Total = 22.04 g
Protein: 21% / 85.00 kcal	Per one serving = 11.02 g
Fat: 60% / 244.00 kcal	
Carbohydrates: 19% / 77.50 kcal	Protein: Total = 21.91 g / p.s. = 10.96 g
Carbohydrates mass fraction: 3.70%	Fat: Total = 28.27 g / p.s. = 14.14 g

6. Hot Blueberry Coconut Cereal

Coconut is always a good choice when it comes to breakfast. It fills your appetite without piling in too many carbs.

Ingredients

For the cereal

- ¼ cup of coconut flour (25g)
- 1 cup of almond milk (240g)
- 10 drops of liquid stevia (10g)
- ¼ cup of ground flaxseed (42g)
- 1 tsp of vanilla extract (4g)
- 1 pinch of salt (1g)
- 1 pinch of cinnamon (1g)

Toppings

- 60 g of blueberries
- 1 oz of shaved coconut (28g)
- 2 tbsp of butter (28g)
- 2 tbsp of pumpkin seeds (8g)

Instructions

- Pour almond milk into a small pot and heat on low.
- Add flaxseed, coconut flour, salt, and cinnamon. Whisk the mixture gently.
- Slowly increase heat until you spot bubbles. Then, add vanilla extract and liquid stevia.
- When the mixture has thickened enough, turn off heat and add toppings.

Servings quantity: 2	Weight:
Energy (calories):	Total = 456.00 g
Total = 870.00 kcal	Per one serving = 228.00 g
Per one serving = 435.00 kcal	**Total carbohydrate:**
Calorie breakdown:	Total = 35.85 g
Protein: 7% / 61.00 kcal	Per one serving = 17.93 g
Fat: 76% / 660.00 kcal	
Carbohydrates: 16% / 137.00 kcal	Protein: Total = 17.41 g / p.s. = 8.71 g
Carbohydrates mass fraction: 7.86%	Fat: Total = 77.48 g / p.s. = 38.74 g

7. Coconut Macadamia Bars

If you're looking for something different, try these coconut macadamia bars. Easy to cook, they're ready in as little as 10 minutes.

Ingredients

- 60 g of macadamia nuts
- ¼ cup of coconut oil (55g)
- 20 drops of stevia (20g)
- 6 tbsp of unsweetened shredded coconut (30g)

Instructions

- Crush the macadamia nuts thoroughly in the blender.
- In a mixing bowl, add coconut oil and shredded coconut. Mix thoroughly.
- Add the macadamia nuts and stevia drops.
- Mix thoroughly then pour the batter into a 9x9 baking dish lined with parchment paper.
- Refrigerate the mixture overnight.

Note: if you want crunchier bars, store them in the freezer.

Servings quantity: -	Weight:
Energy (calories): Total = 1007.00 kcal	Total = 165.00 g
	Total carbohydrate: Total = 13.86 g
Calorie breakdown: Protein: 2% / 20.00 kcal Fat: 93% / 934.00 kcal Carbohydrates: 6% / 56.00 kcal	Protein: Total = 5.75 g
Carbohydrates mass fraction: 8.40%	Fat: Total = 110.00 g

8. Mocha Chia

Quick to make, this is for all those days when you don't feel like cooking an elaborate meal.

Ingredients

- ¾ cup of brewed coffee (159g)
- 1 tbsp almond nut butter (16g)
- ⅔ cup of coconut cream (161g)
- ¼ cup of chia seeds (36g)
- 2 tbsp of granulated butter (28g)
- 1 tsp of vanilla (4g)
- Cinnamon to taste (1g)

Instructions

1. Add all ingredients to mixing bowl and mix thoroughly.
2. Refrigerate overnight.
3. Serve.

Servings quantity: 2	Weight:
Energy (calories): Total = 1024.00 kcal	Total = 424.00 g
Per one serving = 512.00 kcal	Per one serving = 212.00 g
Calorie breakdown:	**Total carbohydrate:**
Protein: 5% / 54.00 kcal	Total = 30.22 g
Fat: 82% / 837.00 kcal	Per one serving = 15.11 g
Carbohydrates: 12% / 122.00 kcal	Protein: Total = 15.62 g / p.s. = 7.81 g
Carbohydrates mass fraction: 7.13%	Fat: Total = 98.79 g / p.s. = 49.40 g

9. Low Carb Blueberry Muffins

Who doesn't like muffins? Here's a quick way to make a keto friendly variety.

Ingredients

- 3 organic eggs, extra large (168g)
- 5 tbsp coconut flour (31g)
- ¼ cup of organic heavy cream (30g)
- ½ cup of frozen blueberries (78g)
- ⅓ cup of erythritol crystals (65g)
- ¼ cup of coconut milk (60g)

Instructions

- Preheat oven to 350.
- Line muffin pan with muffin liners.
- Whisk eggs, cream, and erythritol in a large bowl.
- Add coconut flour to the egg mixture and whisk until smooth.
- Wait until the batter thickens.
- Add frozen blueberries and mix again.
- Spoon the batter into each muffin cup.
- Bake 25 to 30 minutes.

Servings quantity: 6 muffins	**Weight:**
Energy (calories): Total = 738.00 kcal Per one serving = 123.00 kcal	Total = 432.00 g Per one serving = 72.00 g
Calorie breakdown: Protein: 15% / 108.00 kcal Fat: 72% / 533.00 kcal Carbohydrates: 13% / 98.00 kcal	**Total carbohydrate:** Total = 24.50 g Per one serving = 4.08 g Protein: Total = 25.55 g / p.s. = 4.26 g
Carbohydrates mass fraction: 5.67%	Fat: Total = 61.88 g / p.s. = 10.31 g

10.   The Quick Scramble

This is one for quick meal planners and early birds.

Ingredients

- 6 whisked eggs (264g)
- 1 cup of spinach (30g)
- 8 bella mushrooms (baby) (80g)
- 4 slices of deli ham (112g)
- ½ cup of red bell peppers (75g)
- 1 tbsp of coconut oil (14g)
- Salt and pepper (5g)

Instructions

- Thoroughly chop vegetables and ham.
- Melt ½ tbsp of butter in frying pan it.
- sauté the vegetables and ham.
- Pour the whisked eggs into another frying pan. Add ½ tbsp of butter.
- Cook on medium heat while continuously stirring.
- Season eggs with salt and pepper.
- Add the sautéed vegetables and ham to the eggs and mix.

Servings quantity: 2	Weight:
Energy (calories): Total = 731.00 kcal Per one serving = 365.50 kcal	Total = 579.00 g Per one serving = 289.50 g
Calorie breakdown: Protein: 32% / 236.00 kcal Fat: 60% / 437.00 kcal Carbohydrates: 8% / 60.00 kcal	**Total carbohydrate:** Total = 15.98 g Per one serving = 7.99 g
Carbohydrates mass fraction: 2.76%	Protein: Total = 56.08 g / p.s. = 28.04 g Fat: Total = 49.03 g / p.s. = 24.52 g

11.   Sausage Scotch Eggs

There are few things as good for breakfast as traditional scotch eggs; tasty, healthy and fast.

Ingredients

- 1 lb of ground pork (454g)
- 6 medium sized eggs (264g)
- 1 tbsp of homemade gingerbread spice mix (7g)
- 1 tsp of salt (6g)
- 1 tsp black pepper (3g)

Instructions

- Boil the eggs then let cool for ~10 minutes before peeling.
- Preheat oven to 350 F
- Mix gingerbread spice mix, salt, pepper and ground pork in a large bowl.
- For every egg, measure out ⅓ cup of the seasoned ground pork.
- Make patties (similar to hamburger patties) from each lump of pork.
- Place an egg in the center of each patty.
- Fold the pork patties around each egg, fully encasing them as evenly as possible.
- Place them on a baking sheet and bake for 15 to 20 minutes.

Servings quantity: 6 scotch eggs	Weight:
Energy (calories): Total = 1595.00 kcal Per one serving = 265.83 kcal	Total = 733.00 g Per one serving = 122.17 g
Calorie breakdown: Protein: 30% / 473.00 kcal Fat: 69% / 1096.00 kcal Carbohydrates: 2% / 27.00 kcal	**Total carbohydrate:** Total = 8.17 g Per one serving = 1.36 g Protein: Total = 110.74 g / p.s. = 18.46 g
Carbohydrates mass fraction: 1.11%	Fat: Total = 121.54 g / p.s. = 20.26 g

12.   Spicy Egg Frittata

Mmmm… you'll wanna eat a whole lotta this frittata!

Ingredients

- 5 eggs (220g)
- 4 strips of bacon (20g)
- 10–12 cherry tomatoes (190g)
- ½ chopped onion (55g)
- 1-2 minced Serrano peppers (9g)
- 1 chopped green peppers (119g)
- ¼ tsp of black pepper (1g)
- ½ tsp of turmeric (2g)
- Pinch of kosher salt (1g)

Instructions

- Mix eggs, green pepper, Serrano peppers, salt, pepper, and turmeric in a bowl.
- Cook bacon in a cast iron skillet until crisp.
- Remove bacon. Set aside to drain and cool until safe to handle, then crumble thoroughly.
- Pour out excess bacon fat, leaving just enough to coat the bottom of the skillet.
- Add onions then the egg mixture. Stir together.
- Cook for 5 to 6 minutes then add tomatoes and bacon on the top.
- Bake in oven at 350 F for 5 minutes.

Servings quantity: 3	Weight:
Energy (calories):	Total = 617.00 g
Total = 466.00 kcal	Per one serving = 205.67 g
Per one serving = 155.33 kcal	**Total carbohydrate:**
Calorie breakdown:	Total = 22.98 g
Protein: 29% / 137.00 kcal	Per one serving = 7.66 g
Fat: 52% / 244.00 kcal	
Carbohydrates: 18% / 84.00 kcal	Protein: Total = 33.45 g / p.s. = 11.15 g
Carbohydrates mass fraction: 3.72%	Fat: Total = 27.58 g / p.s. = 9.19 g

Chapter 4: Recipes. Keto Snacks

Here are some of the best keto snack recipes. Use these easy munching options between meals.

13. Bacon Wrapped Jalapeno Poppers

Jalapeno poppers are popular worldwide for a reason and they just happen to be perfect for keto.

Ingredients

- 16 fresh jalapenos (224g)
- 16 strips of bacon (80g)
- ¼ cup of cheddar cheese (shredded) (28g)
- 4 oz of cream cheese (113g)
- 1 tsp of salt (6g)
- 1 tsp of paprika (2g)

Instructions

- Preheat oven to 350 F
- Cut the jalapenos in half, lengthwise. Remove the stems, seeds, and inner membrane.
- Mix cream cheese and cheddar cheese together in a bowl.
- Fill each jalapeno half with the cheese mix.
- Wrap each stuffed jalapeno with bacon.
- Place them on a baking dish.
- Bake for 20 to 25 minutes
- Sprinkle salt and paprika to taste.

Servings quantity: 16 jalapeno poppers	**Weight:**
Energy (calories):	Total = 454.00 g
Total = 822.00 kcal	Per one serving = 28.38 g
Per one serving = 51.38 kcal	**Total carbohydrate:**
Calorie breakdown:	Total = 25.85 g
Protein: 11% / 92.00 kcal	Per one serving = 1.62 g
Fat: 77% / 635.00 kcal	
Carbohydrates: 12% / 95.00 kcal	Protein: Total = 24.44 g / p.s. = 1.53 g
Carbohydrates mass fraction: 5.69%	Fat: Total = 73.14 g / p.s. = 4.57 g

14.   Green Bean Fries

If you're really health conscious and looking for a snack you won't have to fuss over, look no further.

Ingredients

- 1 large egg (50g)
- 12 oz of green beans (340g)
- ½ tsp of garlic powder (2g)
- ⅔ cup of grated parmesan (67g)
- ¼ tsp of paprika (1g)
- ¼ tsp black pepper (1g)
- ½ tsp salt (3g)

Instructions

- Preheat oven to 400 F.
- Rinse the green beans, pat dry, and snip the ends.
- In a shallow plate, mix the grated parmesan cheese and seasonings evenly.
- Whisk eggs in a large bowl.
- Dredge the green beans thoroughly in the eggs, letting excess egg drip off.
- Press the green beans onto the cheese mixture.
- Sprinkle more cheese on top.
- Place the beams on a greased baking sheet.
- Bake for 10 minutes until cheese is slightly gold in color.

Servings quantity: 2	Weight:
Energy (calories):	Total = 463.00 g
Total = 436.00 kcal	Per one serving = 231.50 g
Per one serving = 218.00 kcal	**Total carbohydrate:**
Calorie breakdown:	Total = 26.31 g
Protein: 27% / 119.00 kcal	Per one serving = 13.16 g
Fat: 51% / 221.00 kcal	
Carbohydrates: 22% / 97.00 kcal	Protein: Total = 29.55 g / p.s. = 14.78 g
Carbohydrates mass fraction: 5.68%	Fat: Total = 25.08 g / p.s. = 12.54 g

15.   Salted Almond and Coconut Bark

If you like sweet and savory, this one is worth the extra effort.

Ingredients

- ½ cup of coconut butter (109g)
- 100 g of dark chocolate
- ½ cup of almonds (72g)
- ½ tsp of almond extract (4g)
- ½ cup of unsweetened flaked coconut (39g)
- 10 drops of liquid stevia (10g)
- Sea salt to taste (4g)

Instructions

- Preheat the oven to 350F.
- Line a baking sheet with foil. Spread the coconut and almonds on it.
- Toast in the oven for 5 to 8 minutes.
- Stir occasionally to prevent burning.
- After they're thoroughly toasted, set aside to cool.
- Melt the dark chocolate in a double boiler.
- Stir in the coconut butter.
- Add almond extract and liquid stevia. Mix well and set aside.
- Line a baking sheet with parchment paper and pour the chocolate mixture on top.
- Spread evenly using the back of a spoon.
- Sprinkle the roasted almonds and coconut flakes evenly on top and gently press them in
- Sprinkle with sea salt.
- Refrigerate for 1 hour.

Servings quantity: -	**Weight:**
Energy (calories): Total = 2179.00 kcal	Total = 335.00 g
	Total carbohydrate: Total = 77.56 g
Calorie breakdown: Protein: 4% / 88.00 kcal Fat: 80% / 1745.00 kcal Carbohydrates: 14% / 312.00 kcal	Protein: Total = 24.20 g / Fat: Total = 201.83 g /
Carbohydrates mass fraction: 23.15%	

16.   Keto Protein Shake

Shakes are always good for a quick snack.

Ingredients

- 1 tbsp of cocoa powder (5g)
- 1 scoop of chocolate protein powder (30g)
- 1 cup of almond milk (240g)
- 1 tbsp of peanut butter (16g)
- 2 tsp of erythritol (8g)
- 4 ice cubes (120g)
- 1 tbsp of coconut oil (14g)

Instructions

- Mix all the dry ingredients in a large bowl.
- In a blender, add the liquid ingredients and mix briefly.
- Transfer the dry mixture into the blender and mix.
- Add ice cubes and blend thoroughly.

Note: You can choose any main liquid for your shake – water, cream, coconut milk, almond milk, or milk. We recommend sticking with lower carb options.

Servings quantity: 1	Weight:
Energy (calories): Total = 353.00 kcal Per one serving = 353.00 kcal	Total = 433.00 g Per one serving = 433.00 g
Calorie breakdown: Protein: 24% / 86.00 kcal Fat: 65% / 228.00 kcal Carbohydrates: 9% / 31.00 kcal	**Total carbohydrate:** Total = 11.00 g Per one serving = 11.00 g Protein: Total = 22.57 g / p.s. = 22.57 g Fat: Total = 26.49 g / p.s. = 26.49 g
Carbohydrates mass fraction: 2.54%	

17.   Cucumber Boats

This is an exciting and fun recipe, with a presentation suitable for entertaining.

Ingredients

- 1 small cucumber cut in half lengthwise and seeds removed(158g)
- 4 slices of turkey bacon, cooked until crispy, then crumbled (64g)
- 1 6" whole wheat tortilla; low carb (24g)
- 3 oz of softened whipped cream cheese (57g)
- 1 slice of smoked deli turkey, finely diced (28g)
- 1 tbsp of mayonnaise (14g)
- 1 tbsp of grated parmesan cheese (5g)
- ¼ tsp of dried basil (0.3g)
- 1 tbsp of diced pimiento pepper (9g)

Instructions

- Mix cream cheese, dried basil, diced turkey, mayonnaise, parmesan, bacon and pimientos in a medium bowl.
- Using a spoon, hollow out the cucumber halves.
- Spoon the mixture into the cucumber halves.
- Cut the edges off the tortilla to make it square.
- Slice the square in half diagonally, making two triangles.
- Place each cucumber half in the center of a triangle.
- While holding a tortilla triangle wrapped around a cucumber, push a wooden skewer in one side and out the other, forming a 'boat.'
- Place on serving tray.

Servings quantity: 2	Weight:
Energy (calories): Total = 555.00 kcal Per one serving = 277.50 kcal	Total = 359.00 g Per one serving = 179.50 g
	Total carbohydrate: Total = 20.04 g Per one serving = 10.02 g
Calorie breakdown: Protein: 17% / 93.00 kcal Fat: 69% / 384.00 kcal Carbohydrates: 14% / 79.00 kcal	Protein: Total = 23.51 g / p.s. = 11.76 g
Carbohydrates mass fraction: 5.58%	Fat: Total = 43.23 g / p.s. = 21.62 g

18.   Crunchy Kale Chips

Kale chips have managed to gain massive popularity in the last few years. Snack on these healthy and delicious chips during movie time.

Ingredients

- 1 bunch of kale (115g)
- 2 tbsp of parmesan cheese (10g)
- 1 tsp of garlic powder (3g)
- 2 tbsp of olive oil (27g)
- salt and pepper (6g)

Instructions

- Wash kale thoroughly then dry well.
- Cut into smaller pieces as desired.
- In a large mixing bowl, add the kale, olive oil, and seasoning last.
- Gently massage and mix all the ingredients, ensuring both the sides of the kale pieces are coated.
- Space them evenly apart on a cookie sheet.
- Bake at 350 F for 8 to 12 minutes.

Servings quantity: -	Weight:
Energy (calories): Total = 354.00 kcal	Total = 161.00 g
	Total carbohydrate: Total = 14.58 g
Calorie breakdown: Protein: 8% / 30.00 kcal Fat: 77% / 273.00 kcal Carbohydrates: 15% / 52.00 kcal	Protein: Total = 9.53 g
Carbohydrates mass fraction: 9.06%	Fat: Total = 30.92 g

19.   Bulletproof Coffee

Isn't coffee something we're all addicted to? Here's a keto twist you might like.

Ingredients

- 2 tbsp of coffee grounds (10g)
- 1 tbsp of coconut oil (14g)
- 1 cup of water (235g)
- 1 tbsp of grass fed butter (14g)

Instructions

- Use your own preferred method of making a cup of coffee.
- Pour the coffee into a blender.
- Add butter and coconut oil.
- Blend thoroughly.
- Feel free to add ingredients like cinnamon, nutmeg, whipped cream, and stevia.

Servings quantity: 1	Weight:
Energy (calories): Total = 221.00 kcal Per one serving = 221.00 kcal	Total = 273.00 g Per one serving = 273.00 g
Calorie breakdown: Protein: 1% / 2.00 kcal Fat: 99% / 219.00 kcal Carbohydrates: 0% / 1.00 kcal	**Total carbohydrate:** Total = 0.33 g Per one serving = 0.33 g Protein: Total = 0.41 g / p.s. = 0.41 g Fat: Total = 25.17 g / p.s. = 25.17 g
Carbohydrates mass fraction: 0.12%	

20.   Easy Guacamole

A summertime staple, this one is quick and zesty.

Ingredients

- 2 avocados (402g)
- 6 grape tomatoes (102g)
- ¼ cup of diced red onion (40g)
- 1 juiced lime (44g)
- 1 garlic clove (3g)
- 1 tbsp of olive oil (14g)
- Fresh cilantro (10g)
- ¼ tsp of salt (1.5g)
- ⅛ tsp of crushed red pepper (0.2g)
- ⅛ tsp of black pepper (0.3g)

Instructions

- Peel and pit the avocados.
- Mash the avocados in a mixing bowl.
- Dice the grape tomatoes and red onions and dice them evenly.
- Add the diced tomatoes and onions to the avocados.
- Add the olive oil.
- Use a garlic press to squeeze the clove into the mixture.
- Mix well.
- Add the lime juice and cilantro and mix again.
- Finally, season with salt, pepper, and crushed red pepper.

Servings quantity: 2	**Weight:**
Energy (calories):	Total = 617.00 g
Total = 816.00 kcal	Per one serving = 308.50 g
Per one serving = 408.00 kcal	**Total carbohydrate:**
Calorie breakdown:	Total = 47.34 g
Protein: 4% / 32.00 kcal	Per one serving = 23.67 g
Fat: 75% / 616.00 kcal	
Carbohydrates: 21% / 168.00 kcal	Protein: Total = 10.00 g / p.s. = 5.00 g
Carbohydrates mass fraction: 7,67%	Fat: Total = 72.80 g / p.s. = 36.40 g

21.   Coconut Butter Cups

Seriously decadent sweet goodness.

Ingredients

- 2 tbsp of coconut butter (27g)
- 2 tbsp of erythritol (25g)
- 4 tbsp of cocoa powder (22g)
- 4 tsp of coconut powder (6g)
- 4 tbsp of coconut oil (54g)
- 1 pinch of salt (1g)

Instructions

1. Mix coconut oil, erythritol and cocoa powder in a bowl until smooth.
2. Add salt and stir to distribute.
3. Coat 4 cups of a silicone cupcake mold with coconut butter.
4. Pour the chocolate mixture into the cupcake molds. Make to a point to tilt and turn the mold to entirely coat each cup.
5. Freeze for 5 minutes.
6. When the bottom layer has hardened completely, pour a tsp of coconut oil in each mold.
7. Place it in the freezer for a few more minutes.
8. Take the leftover chocolate mixture and cover gelled coconut oil.
9. Freeze again for 5 minutes.
10. Pop from molds to serve.

Servings quantity: 4 coconut butter cups	**Weight:**
Energy (calories): Total = 800 kcal Per one coconut butter cup = 200 kcal	Total = 135 g Per one coconut butter cup = 33.75 g
Calorie breakdown: Protein: 1% / 9 kcal Fat: 95% / 759 kcal Carbohydrates: 4% / 32 kcal	**Total carbohydrate:** Total = 15.31 g Per one serving = 3.83 g
Carbohydrates mass fraction: 11.34%	**Protein:** Total = 4.32g / p.s. = 1.08g **Fat:** Total = 88.3g / p.s. = 22.08g

22.   Protein Shake

What's better than a protein shake to quell your hunger and provide long-lasting energy for the day's activities?

Ingredients

- 1 scoop of chocolate protein powder (30g)
- 3/4 cup of coconut milk (180g)
- 1 tbsp of peanut butter (16g)
- 2 tsp of erythritol (8g)
- 6 ice cubes (180g)
- 1 tbsp of cocoa powder (5g)
- 1 tbsp of coconut oil (14g)

Instructions

- Mix all the dry ingredients in a blender.
- Add all the wet ingredients and mix.
- Add ice cubes and blend until smooth.

Note: You can choose any main liquid for your shake – water, cream, coconut milk, almond milk, and cashew milk are all good options.

Servings quantity: 1	Weight:
Energy (calories): Total = 756.00 kcal	Total = 433.00 g Per one serving = 433.00 g
Per one serving = 756.00 kcal	**Total carbohydrate:**
Calorie breakdown: Protein: 13% / 96.00 kcal	Total = 22.36 g Per one serving = 22.36 g
Fat: 75% / 564.00 kcal	
Carbohydrates: 11% / 83.00 kcal	Protein: Total = 25.69 g / p.s. = 25.69 g
Carbohydrates mass fraction: 5.16%	Fat: Total = 66.90 g / p.s. = 66.90 g

23.   Sugar Free Peanut Butter Fudge

We know that merely mentioning dessert might elicit serious food cravings, but this recipe is completely sugar free and adheres to ketogenic recommendations as well.

Ingredients

- ¼ cup of unsweetened vanilla almond milk (60g)
- 1 cup of unsweetened peanut butter (258g)
- 1 cup of coconut oil (218g)

Instructions

- In a microwave safe bowl, combine peanut butter and coconut oil. Heat gently to soften.
- Put this mixture in the blender.
- Add the almond milk and blend thoroughly.
- Pour the mix into a parchment lined pan.
- Refrigerate for 2 hours.

Servings quantity: -	Weight:
Energy (calories): Total = 3400.00 kcal	Total = 534.00 g
	Total carbohydrate: Total = 56.39 g
Calorie breakdown: Protein: 6% / 215.00 kcal Fat: 87% / 2955.00 kcal Carbohydrates: 7% / 228.25 kcal	Protein: Total = 61.82 g /
Carbohydrates mass fraction: 10.56%	Fat: Total = 346.49 g /

24.   Antipasto Kebabs

Based on your appetite, these can be used as snacks or lunch.

Ingredients

- spanish queen green olives
- baby heirloom tomatoes
- kalamata olives
- marinated artichoke hearts
- marinated fresh mozzarella balls
- sliced salami
- pepperoncinis

Instructions

- Take all the ingredients and thread them onto skewers in an alternating fashion.
- That's it. Serve.

Servings quantity, calories, carbs and other values: vary.

Chapter 5: Recipes. Ketogenic Lunch

Now that we've dealt with breakfast and snacks, it's time for some healthy yet lip-smacking lunch recipes.

25. Paleo Burrito Bowl Recipe

This is an amazingly healthy choice for lunch and takes less than 20 minutes to prep.

Ingredients

- 1 large chopped onion (110g)
- 4 chopped roma tomatoes (248g)
- 1 cup of sliced black olives (135g)
- 2 cups of leftover taco spiced beef (450g)
- 1 sliced ripe avocado (201g)
- 2 tbsp of coconut oil (27g)
- 3 cups of riced cauliflower (321g)
- 5 cups of shredded lettuce (275g)
- diced cilantro (9g)
- 1 cup of salsa (260g)

Instructions

- In a pan, sauté olives, onion, and cauliflower in the coconut oil.
- Add the taco meat along with the tomatoes. Cook until evenly hot.
- Serve along with shredded lettuce. Top with salsa, diced cilantro, and avocado.

Servings quantity: 8	**Weight:**
Energy (calories): Total = 1538 kcal Per one serving = 384.5 kcal	Total = 2036 g Per one serving = 254.5 g
Calorie breakdown: Protein: 30% / 455 kcal Fat: 50% / 772 kcal Carbohydrates: 20% / 311 kcal	**Total carbohydrate:** Total = 86.08 g Per one serving = 10.76 g
Carbohydrates mass fraction: 4.23%	**Protein:** Total = 121.22g / p.s. = 15.15g **Fat:** Total = 90.1g / p.s. = 11.26g

26.	**Rosemary Balsamic Chicken Liver Pate**

This is for those days when you want a filling lunch.

Ingredients

- 1 pound of chicken liver (454g)
- 1 cup of chopped leek; green parts (89g)
- 1 tbsp of apple cider vinegar (15g)
- 2 -3 tbsp of balsamic vinegar (40g)
- ¼ cup of coconut oil (55g)
- 1 sprig of fresh rosemary (removed from the stem) (3g)
- 1 tsp of freshly ground pepper (3g)
- ½ tsp of sea salt (3g)
- filtered water

Instructions

- Using a glass baking dish, marinate the liver in a water and apple cider vinegar solution for 12 to 24 hours.
- When you feel that it's ready, drain the liver and place it in a cast iron pan along with coconut oil, rosemary, leeks, and salt.
- Cover and cook on medium low heat for 10 minutes.
- Remove from heat and set aside for 5 minutes.
- Transfer the liver and juices to your blender.
- Add balsamic vinegar and ground pepper.
- Blend until very smooth.
- Spoon the mixture into a shallow sealable container.
- Seal container and store in the fridge for 2 to 3 days.

Servings quantity: -	Weight:
Energy (calories): Total = 1113 kcal	Total = 661 g
Calorie breakdown: Protein: 30% / 333 kcal Fat: 61% / 672 kcal Carbohydrates: 9% / 97 kcal	**Total carbohydrate:** Total = 25.33 g **Protein:** Total = 78.68 g
Carbohydrates mass fraction: 3.83%	**Fat:** Total = 76.95 g

27.   Paleo Stuffed Avocado

Tasty, creamy, and chock full of healthy fats, avocados are virtually the poster food for keto.

Ingredients

- 1 large avocado (201g)
- 1 medium spring onion (15g)
- 1 tin of drained sardines (92g)
- 1 tbsp of fresh lemon juice (15g)
- 1 tbsp of mayonnaise (14g)
- ¼ tsp of salt (2g)
- ¼ tsp of turmeric powder (1g)

Instructions

- Halve and pit avocado.
- Drain the sardines and place in mixing bowl.
- Break them into smaller pieces.
- Scoop out the middle portion of the avocado halves, leaving ½ to 1 inch of flesh.
- Slice the spring onion evenly and add to the sardines.
- Add freshly grated turmeric.
- Add mayonnaise and mix it thoroughly
- Add the scooped avocado flesh and mash thoroughly.
- Squeeze the lemon juice and add.
- Add salt and mash to distribute evenly.
- Scoop the mixture into the avocado halves and serve.

Servings quantity: 2	Weight:
Energy (calories): Total = 617 kcal Per one serving = 308.5 kcal	Total = 339 g Per one serving = 169.5 g
Calorie breakdown: Protein: 18% / 112 kcal Fat: 70% / 435 kcal Carbohydrates: 11% / 71 kcal	**Total carbohydrate:** Total = 19.92 g Per one serving = 9.96 g
Carbohydrates mass fraction: 5.88%	**Protein:** Total = 27.21g / p.s. = 13.61g **Fat:** Total = 50.42g / p.s. = 25.21g

28.   Low Carb Salmon and Avocado Sushi

If you're a sushi lover, we've included this recipe just for you.

Ingredients

- 500 g of riced cauliflower
- 50 g of smoked salmon
- 1 sliced avocado (200g)
- 4 nori papers (10g)
- 2 tbsp of softened butter (28g)
- 4 tbsp whipped cream cheese (40g)
- 1 tbsp of rice vinegar (15g)

Instructions

- Heat a pan on heat and add cauliflower rice along with butter.
- sauté for 10 to 15 minutes.
- Let it rest until cool.
- Completely coat the nori paper with a layer of cream cheese.
- Stir rice vinegar into the cauliflower mixture.
- Pat the rice mixture onto the cream cheese layer.
- Place salmon and avocado slices on top, at and parallel to the edge.
- Roll like sushi and serve.

Servings quantity: 4	Weight:
Energy (calories): Total = 878 kcal Per one serving = 219.5 kcal	Total = 844 g Per one serving = 211 g
Calorie breakdown: Protein: 11% / 95 kcal Fat: 69% / 604 kcal Carbohydrates: 20% / 176 kcal	**Total carbohydrate:** Total = 49.02 g Per one serving = 12.26 g
Carbohydrates mass fraction: 5.8%	**Protein:** Total = 28.56g / p.s. = 7.14g **Fat:** Total = 70.16g / p.s. = 17.54g

29.   Low Carb Pizza

Yes, you read correctly. You can even have pizza while on a ketogenic diet. All the more reasons to stick with it, yeah?

Ingredients

- 1 medium head of cauliflower (590g)
- 1 cup of chia seeds (144g)
- 1 cup of water (237g)
- 3 tbsp of olive oil (41g)
- 1 tsp of sea salt (6g)
- ½ cup of cream cheese (120g)
- 2 cloves of peeled garlic (6g)
- ½ cup of grated parmesan cheese (50g)
- ½ cup of heavy cream (60g)

Instructions

- Remove all the cauliflower florets from the stem.
- Using a food processor, chop them into smaller pieces.
- Grind the chia seeds into flour.
- Combine the chia flour, chopped cauliflower, water, olive oil, and salt.
- Mix well until you get a smooth dough.
- Let rest for 20 minutes.
- Coat a cookie sheet with olive oil.
- Spread the dough on the cookie sheet.
- Bake at 200 F for 1 hour.
- The crust should be cooked thoroughly. If not, keep a close watch while baking it longer.
- When the crust is ready, remove from oven.
- Preheat oven to 400 F.
- Mix the cheese cream and garlic until smooth.
- Spread it on the pizza crust.
- Bake at 400 F for 10 minutes.

Note: You can add keto friendly vegetable toppings as desired.

Servings quantity: 5	Weight:
Energy (calories): Total = 1985 kcal Per one serving = 397 kcal	Total = 1252 g Per one serving = 250.4 g
Calorie breakdown: Protein: 11% / 99 kcal Fat: 71% / 648 kcal Carbohydrates: 18% / 159 kcal	Total carbohydrate: Total = 104.69 g Per one serving = 20.94 g
Carbohydrates mass fraction: 8.36%	Protein: Total = 57.81g / p.s. = 11.56g Fat: Total = 162.28g / p.s. = 32.46g

30.   Pork and Egg Pie

When you absolutely love bacon, this recipe is everything you'll ever need.

Ingredients

- 6 large slices of unsmoked bacon (156g)
- 1 recipe for Low Carb Pie Crust (320g)
- 1 medium red onion, finely chopped (110g)
- 4 large eggs (200g)
- 350 g of diced pork loin
- ¼ cup freshly chopped spring onion (25g)
- 2 tbsp of lard (26g)
- 2 cloves of crushed garlic (6g)
- ½ cup of full-fat cream cheese (116g)
- 1 cup of grated cheddar cheese (113g)
- ½ tsp salt (3g)
- freshly ground black pepper (6g)

Instructions

- Make the pie crust using your own recipe. Ideally, we recommend making one regular crust, but 8 mini pie crusts are fine too.
- Place baking paper on top and weigh the dough down with the help of ceramic baking beans.
- Place in the oven and bake for 12 to 15 minutes.
- Finely chop 2 slices of uncooked bacon.
- Place in a pan with garlic.
- Stirring continuously, cook for 5 to 7 minutes.
- Add the remaining bacon slices and cook 5 more minutes.
- Dice the pork loin and add it to the pan.
- Cook over medium heat until browned on all sides.
- Remove let cool.
- Preheat oven to 400 F.
- Combine meat with cream cheese, salt, and pepper.
- Crack eggs in a large mixing bowl.
- Add grated cheddar cheese and mix well.
- Add spring onion and mix again.
- Add meat and cream cheese mixture to the bowl and combine thoroughly.

- Spoon the entire mixture evenly into the pie crust.
- Place pie in oven and bake for 25 minutes.

Servings quantity: 8	**Weight:** Total = 1430 g Per one serving = 178.75g
Energy (calories): Total = 3663 kcal Per one serving = 457.9 kcal	
Calorie breakdown: Protein: 20% / 732 kcal Fat: 75% / 2748 kcal Carbohydrates: 5% / 183 kcal	**Total carbohydrate:** Total = 79.72 g Per one serving = 9.97g
Carbohydrates mass fraction: 5.57%	**Protein:** Total = 172.72g / p.s. = 21.59g **Fat:** Total = 306.17g / p.s. = 38.27g

31.   Grilled Tomatoes with Apricot Jam

This can be used either as a snack or for lunch.

Ingredients

- 6 medium sized tomatoes (738g)
- 2 tsp of dried oregano (2g)
- 1 ½ oz of watercress for garnishing (43g)
- 3 tsp of sugar free apricot jam (18g)
- 3 ½ oz of grated Gouda cheese (99g)
- 1 tbsp of olive oil (14g)
- salt and pepper (12g)

Instructions

- Preheat oven to 350 F.
- Cut the tomatoes into halves and place cut side up on a lightly greased baking tray.
- Spread jam on each of the tomato slices.
- Sprinkle oregano on top.
- Grate the cheese on top
- Bake for 25 minutes or until the cheese turns golden.
- Drizzle with olive oil and top with black pepper.
- Garnish with watercress.

Servings quantity: 4 (3 tomato halves per serving)	Weight:
Energy (calories): Total = 656 kcal Per one serving = 164 kcal	Total = 925 g Per one serving = 231g
Calorie breakdown: Protein: 19% / 126 kcal Fat: 57% / 374 kcal Carbohydrates: 24% / 155 kcal	**Total carbohydrate:** Total = 43.24g Per one serving = 10.81g
Carbohydrates mass fraction: 4.7%	**Protein:** Total = 33.1g / p.s. = 8.28g **Fat:** Total = 42.56g / p.s. = 10.64g

32.   Brie and Apple Crepes

This dish scores points for presentation too.

Ingredients

For the crepe batter

- 4 oz of cream cheese (113g)
- ½ tsp of baking soda (2g)
- 4 large eggs (200g)
- ¼ tsp of salt (2g)

For the toppings

- 2 oz of chopped pecans (57g)
- 1 small sweet apple (150g)
- 1 tbsp of unsalted butter (14g)
- 4 oz of brie cheese (113g)
- ¼ tsp of cinnamon (1g)
- fresh mint leaves

Instructions

- Put all the batter ingredients in a blender and blend until smooth.
- Add a small amount of unsalted butter to a non-stick pan and heat on medium.
- Ladle some of the crepe butter into the pan. Swirl to spread evenly into a thin layer.
- Cook until the top seems to have dried, then flip it gently and cook the other side for few seconds.
- Repeat the last 2 steps until you have about 1 crepe left.
- On a plate, layer them one on the top of the other on a plate and start working on the toppings.
- Melt butter in a small pan.
- Toast the chopped pecans. Sprinkle cinnamon on top and mix
- Transfer pecans to a plate and let cool.
- Make apple and brie cheese slices.
- Arrange the apple slices and brie on a crepe and top with roasted pecans.
- Repeat for all the crepes.
- Garnish with mint.

Servings quantity: 2	**Weight:**
Energy (calories): Total = 1593 kcal Per one serving = 796.5 kcal	Total = 652 g Per one serving = 326g
Calorie breakdown: Protein: 16% / 260 kcal Fat: 75% / 1202 kcal Carbohydrates: 8% / 133 kcal	**Total carbohydrate:** Total = 35.57g Per one serving = 17.79g
Carbohydrates mass fraction: 5.45%	**Protein:** Total = 61.45g / p.s. = 30.73g **Fat:** Total = 138.02g / p.s. = 69.01g

33.   Coleslaw Stuffed Keto Wraps

This is a great recipe for anyone who loves to cook.

Ingredients

For coleslaw

- ½ cup of diced green onions (36g)
- 3 cups of thinly sliced red cabbage (267g)
- 2 tsp of apple cider vinegar (10g)
- ¾ cup of mayonnaise (180g)
- ¼ tsp of sea salt (2g)

Wraps and filling

- 16 collard leaves with stems removed (240g)
- ⅓ cup of packed alfalfa sprouts (11g)
- 1 lb of regular gourd meat (454g)

Instructions

- Mix all coleslaw ingredients in a large bowl, ensuring everything is well coated.
- When you have removed the stems, each collard leaf should have a missing strip from the base to almost midway up the leaf.
- Place the first collard leaf on a clean surface
- Orient the leaf so the base and missing stem strip are further away from you.
- Place a spoonful of coleslaw toward the top edge of the leaf. Put a spoonful of meat on top of that and top with sprouts.
- Roll the top of the leaf over the mixture then begin folding the sides in to prevent the filling from spilling out.
- Continue rolling and try to overlap the edges where the strip is missing.
- When complete, insert 1 or 2 toothpicks to prevent unraveling.
- Repeat with the leftover leaves and filling.
- Divide the wraps into 4 servings of 4 wraps each.

Servings quantity: 4	Weight:
Energy (calories): Total = 817 kcal Per one serving = 204.25 kcal	Total = 1200 g Per one serving = 300g
Calorie breakdown: Protein: 10% / 79 kcal Fat: 66% / 534 kcal Carbohydrates: 25% / 202 kcal	**Total carbohydrate:** Total = 55.93g Per one serving = 13.98g
Carbohydrates mass fraction: 4.66%	**Protein:** Total = 25.37g / p.s. = 6.34g **Fat:** Total = 59.45g / p.s. = 14.86g

34.   Ranch Chicken and Veggies

This is a classic recipe everyone enjoys.

Ingredients

- 2 large, thick boneless chicken breasts (580g)
- 300g assorted veggies cut into 1-inch pieces
- 3 tablespoons melted butter (43g)
- ½ tsp onion powder (1g)
- ½ tsp dried chives
- ½ tsp dried parsley
- ½ tsp garlic powder (2g)
- ½ tsp dried dill (1g)
- a pinch of black pepper (1g)
- ½ tsp sea salt (3g)

Instructions

- Preheat oven to 400 F.
- Line a large sheet pan with parchment paper.
- Place all chicken and veggies on it.
- In a small bowl, mix the dill, garlic powder, dried parsley, chives, onion powder, salt, and pepper.
- Sprinkle this mixture over the chicken and veggies.
- Melt butter in a small microwave safe bowl.
- Drizzle on top of chicken and veggies.
- Bake for 35 to 40 minutes.

Servings quantity: 4	Weight:
Energy (calories): Total = 1310 kcal Per one serving = 327.5 kcal	Total = 930 g Per one serving = 232.5g
Calorie breakdown: Protein: 10% / 79 kcal Fat: 66% / 534 kcal Carbohydrates: 25% / 202 kcal	**Total carbohydrate:** Total = 16.39g Per one serving = 4.1g
Carbohydrates mass fraction: 1.76%	**Protein:** Total = 178.16g / p.s. = 44.54g **Fat:** Total = 57.1g / p.s. = 14.28g

35.   Rainbow Stir Fry

Easily made and good eatin'!

Ingredients

- 1 cup cooked chicken (140g)
- 6 peeled carrots (366g)
- ½ small diced onion (35g)
- 2 cloves of minced garlic (6g)
- 3-4 tbsp of coconut aminos (52g)
- 1-2 cups of green beans (230g)
- ¼ cup of real butter (57g)
- sea salt (6g)
- pepper (6g)

Instructions

- In a large pan, aauté the onions in butter for 5 minutes.
- Add a bit of sea salt.
- Add garlic and cook for another minute.
- Add green beans, carrots, coconut aminos, and chicken. Cook on medium heat until the vegetables are cooked through.
- Add salt and pepper to taste.

Servings quantity: 4	Weight:
Energy (calories): Total = 952 kcal Per one serving = 238 kcal	Total = 897 g Per one serving = 224.25g
Calorie breakdown: Protein: 18% / 169 kcal Fat: 61% / 582 kcal Carbohydrates: 21% / 203 kcal	**Total carbohydrate:** Total = 54.1g Per one serving = 13.53g
Carbohydrates mass fraction: 6.03%	**Protein:** Total = 42.4g / p.s. = 10.6g **Fat:** Total = 65.85g / p.s. = 16.46g

36.   Creamy Chicken Casserole

Yet another yummy recipe for all the chicken lovers out there.

Ingredients

- 2 lbs chicken thighs (907g)
- 2 tbsp green pesto (30g)
- ⅔ lb cauliflower (304g)
- 4 oz. cherry tomatoes (113g)
- 7 oz. shredded cheese (199g)
- 3 tbsp butter (43g)
- 1¼ cups heavy whipping cream (150g)
- 1 leek (89g)
- ½ tbsp lemon juice (8g)
- salt and pepper (12g)

Instructions

- Preheat oven to 400 F.
- Mix the cream with pesto and lemon juice. Add salt and pepper to taste
- Season the chicken with salt and pepper.
- Fry them in butter until lightly golden.
- Place the chicken in a baking dish and pour the cream mixture on top.
- Chop the leek, cherry tomatoes, and cauliflower.
- Top the chicken with this mixture.
- Sprinkle cheese on top and bake for 30 minutes.

Servings quantity: 8	Weight:
Energy (calories): Total = 3907 kcal Per one serving = 488.38 kcal	Total = 2018g Per one serving = 252.25g
Calorie breakdown: Protein: 18% / 169 kcal Fat: 61% / 582 kcal Carbohydrates: 21% / 203 kcal	**Total carbohydrate:** Total = 45.58g Per one serving = 5.69g
Carbohydrates mass fraction: 2.26%	**Protein:** Total = 213.85g / p.s. = 26.73g **Fat:** Total = 320g / p.s. = 40g

37.   Mushroom Omelette

If you have a thing for mushrooms, omelettes or better yet, both, try this recipe now!

Ingredients

- ¼ yellow onion (28g)
- 3 eggs (132g)
- 2 – 3 mushrooms (45g)
- ⅞ oz. shredded cheese (25g)
- ⅞ oz. Butter (25g)
- salt and pepper

Instructions

- Crack eggs into a mixing bowl. Add a pinch of salt and pepper.
- Whisk the eggs until smooth.
- Melt butter in a frying pan.
- Pour in the eggs.
- When the bottom has skimmed and the middle gelled, sprinkle some cheese on top.
- Add mushrooms and onions.
- Carefully ease the edges of the omelette and fold it in half.
- When the omelette has turned golden brown underneath, remove the pan from the heat source and slide the omelette onto a plate.

Servings quantity: 1	Weight:
Energy (calories): Total = 481 kcal	Total = 254g
Calorie breakdown: Protein: 22% / 104 kcal Fat: 74% / 359 kcal Carbohydrates: 4% / 19 kcal	**Total carbohydrate:** Total = 5.17g **Protein:** Total = 24.58g
Carbohydrates mass fraction: 2.04%	**Fat:** Total = 40.47g

38.   Garlic Chicken

Another tasty and simple quick fix recipe.

Ingredients

- 8 tbsp of finely chopped fresh parsley (30g)
- 2½ lbs chicken thighs (1134g)
- 5 – 10 of sliced garlic cloves (23g)
- 1 tbsp of lemon juice (15g)
- 2 tbsp of olive oil (27g)
- 4 tbsp of butter (57g)

Instructions

- Preheat oven to 400 F.
- Grease a baking pan with butter and place the chicken pieces on it.
- Sprinkle salt and pepper as desired.
- Sprinkle garlic and parsley over the chicken pieces.
- Drizzle lemon juice and olive oil on top.
- Bake until chicken is golden in color, and the garlic is lightly toasted.

Servings quantity: 5	Weight:
Energy (calories): Total = 3200 kcal Per one serving = 640 kcal	Total = 1286g Per one serving = 257.2g
Calorie breakdown: Protein: 25% / 808 kcal Fat: 73% / 2346 kcal Carbohydrates: 2% / 49 kcal	**Total carbohydrate:** Total = 13.29g Per one serving = 2.66g
Carbohydrates mass fraction: 1.03%	**Protein:** Total = 190.21g / p.s. = 38.04g **Fat:** Total = 261.82g / p.s. = 52.36g

39.   Smoky Tuna Pickle Boats

Here's a recipe for when you need a packable lunch.

Ingredients

- 6 large whole dill pickles (810g)
- (1) 6 oz can of smoked tuna (170g)
- (2) 6 oz cans of albacore tuna (340g)
- ¼ tsp garlic powder (1g)
- ½ tsp onion powder (1g)
- ⅓ cup sugar free mayonnaise (79g)
- ¼ tsp ground black pepper (1g)

Instructions

- Except for the pickles, mix all the ingredients in a mid-sized bowl.
- Cut the pickles lengthwise into halves.
- Gently scoop out the seeds.
- Spoon the tuna salad mixture into the pickle halves.
- Chill before serving.

Servings quantity: 12	Weight:
Energy (calories): Total = 800 kcal Per one serving = 66.67 kcal	Total = 1402g Per one serving = 116.83g
Calorie breakdown: Protein: 53% / 426 kcal Fat: 36% / 291 kcal Carbohydrates: 11% / 87 kcal	**Total carbohydrate:** Total = 23.92g Per one serving = 1.99g
Carbohydrates mass fraction: 1.71%	**Protein:** Total = 108.29g / p.s. = 9.02g **Fat:** Total = 32.55g / p.s. = 2.71g

40.   Rutabaga Fritters with Avocado

This can be used as a lunch or dinner recipe.

Ingredients

For rutabaga fritters

- 4 eggs (176g)
- 1 lb rutabaga (454g)
- 3 tbsp coconut flour (16g)
- ½ lb halloo cheese (227g)
- 4 oz. butter (113g)
- ½ cup turmeric (75g)
- 1 tsp salt (6g)
- ¼ tsp pepper (1g)

For ranch mayonnaise

- 1 cup of mayonnaise (240g)
- 1 tbsp of ranch seasoning (9g)

For serving

- ⅓ lb of leafy greens (150g)
- 4 avocados (804g)

Instructions

- Preheat oven to 250 F.
- Rinse the rutabaga and peel.
- Grate the rutabaga and cheese into a bowl.
- In a large bowl, combine the eggs, rutabaga, cheese, coconut flour, salt, pepper and turmeric. Let it sit for 5 minutes so the flour is fully saturated.
- Heat butter over medium heat in a large frying pan.
- Make 12 patties out of the batter.
- Fry each patty for 3 to 5 minutes on one side. When done, flip to cook the other side.
- Serve with green salad, sliced avocado and the ranch flavoured mayonnaise.

Servings quantity: 6	Weight:
Energy (calories): Total = 4497 kcal Per one serving = 749.5 kcal	Total = 2207g Per one serving = 367.83g
Calorie breakdown: Protein: 11% / 491 kcal Fat: 73% / 3302 kcal Carbohydrates: 16% / 701 kcal	**Total carbohydrate:** Total = 186.37g Per one serving = 31.06g
Carbohydrates mass fraction: 8.44%	**Protein:** Total = 124.12g / p.s. = 20.69g **Fat:** Total = 379.42g / p.s. = 63.24g

Chapter 6: Recipes. Keto Dinner

And the moment we've all been waiting for… dinner!

41.   Coconut Chicken Fingers

Tasty tender tropical goodness!

Ingredients

- 1 egg (44g)
- 1 pound of boneless, skinless chicken tenders (454g)
- ⅛ tsp of cinnamon
- 1 cup unsweetened shredded coconut (80g)
- ½ cup cashew flour (69g)
- ¼ tsp garlic powder (1g)
- ¼ tsp salt (2g)
- ¼ tsp pepper (1g)

Instructions

- Preheat oven to 375 F.
- Line a baking sheet with parchment paper.
- Beat the egg in a bowl and set aside.
- In another bowl, add coconut flakes and spices, along with the cashew flour.
- Dip the chicken tenders in the egg then dredge in the flour mixture.
- Arrange the tenders on the baking sheet, spaced evenly.
- Bake for 15 to 20 minutes.

Servings quantity: 2	Weight:
Energy (calories): Total = 1248 kcal Per one serving = 624 kcal	Total = 649g Per one serving = 324.5g
Calorie breakdown: Protein: 37% / 464 kcal Fat: 51% / 638 kcal Carbohydrates: 12% / 146 kcal	**Total carbohydrate:** Total = 36.16g Per one serving = 18.08g
Carbohydrates mass fraction: 5.57 %	**Protein:** Total = 111.12g / p.s. = 55.56g **Fat:** Total = 75g / p.s. = 37.5g

42. Beef and liver burger recipe

Count on making this a permanent part of your repertoire, because this burger is definitely that yummy.

Ingredients

- ¼ lb chicken livers (113g)
- 1 ¼ lbs ground beef (567g)
- ½ medium peeled red onion (55g)
- 1 tsp poultry seasoning (2g)
- 1 ½ tsp coriander (1g)
- 1 tsp sea salt (6g)
- 1 tsp ground black pepper (3g)

Instructions

- In a food processor, add the red onion and chicken livers.
- Pulse it until you get a smooth paste.
- Add the ground beef and all the spices.
- Pulse the food processor until the texture is not quite smooth.
- Shape this mixture into four patties, 4" in diameter.
- Grill to your liking!

Servings quantity: 4	Weight:
Energy (calories): Total = 1612 kcal Per one serving = 403 kcal	Total = 747g Per one serving = 186.75g
Calorie breakdown: Protein: 31% / 501 kcal Fat: 67% / 1075 kcal Carbohydrates: 2% / 34 kcal	**Total carbohydrate:** Total = 9.27g Per one serving = 2.32g
Carbohydrates mass fraction: 1.24 %	**Protein:** Total = 117.79g / p.s. = 29.45g **Fat:** Total = 119.18g / p.s. = 29.80g

43.   Bacon Burgers

Simple yet heavenly marriage of beef and bacon. Need we say more?

Ingredients

- 2 eggs (88g)
- 4 slices of uncooked bacon (104g)
- 2 lb of ground beef (907g)
- ½ tsp of chipotle chili powder (1g)
- Salt (9g)

Instructions

- Chop the bacon into a variety of sizes, from medium to minced.
- Add the bacon to a large bowl, along with the chili pepper and a touch of salt.
- Mix thoroughly.
- Add the ground beef.
- Mix thoroughly while salting to taste.
- Form into patties.
- Heat the grill to 450 F.
- Grill the patties over direct heat for 2 per side.
- Move them to indirect heat and grill for another 3 to 4 minutes per side.

Servings quantity: 6	Weight:
Energy (calories): Total = 2857 kcal Per one serving = 476.17 kcal	Total = 1110g Per one serving = 185g
Calorie breakdown: Protein: 27% / 776 kcal Fat: 73% / 2081 kcal Carbohydrates: 0.2% / 7 kcal	**Total carbohydrate:** Total = 2.19g Per one serving =0.37g
Carbohydrates mass fraction: 0.2 %	**Protein:** Total = 180.04g / p.s. = 30g **Fat:** Total = 230.85g / p.s. = 38.46g

44. Garlic Roasted Shrimp with Zucchini Pasta

Pasta and keto aren't common bedfellows, but variety is the spice of life. So enjoy this one no more than once a week.

Ingredients

- 8 oz peeled shrimp (227g)
- 2 medium sized boxes of zucchini rotini (640g)
- 1 lemon zest (58g)
- 2 tbsp of melted butter (28g)
- 2 cloves of minced garlic (6g)
- 2 tbsp olive oil (27g)
- ¼ tsp salt (2g)
- fresh ground pepper to taste (2g)

Instructions

- Preheat oven to 400 F.
- In a baking dish, mix all the ingredients except for the pasta.
- Bake for 8 to 10 minutes, stirring the mixture thoroughly about halfway.
- In a large pot, bring water to a boil and add the pasta.
- Cook until al dente and drain well.
- Ensure the shrimp has been cooked thoroughly.
- When complete, add the pasta. Toss it and serve.

Servings quantity: 4	Weight:
Energy (calories): Total = 1347 kcal Per one serving = 336.75 kcal	Total = 1030g Per one serving = 257.5g
Calorie breakdown: Protein: 24% / 327 kcal Fat: 48% / 647 kcal Carbohydrates: 28% / 371 kcal	**Total carbohydrate:** Total = 93.95g Per one serving = 23.48g
Carbohydrates mass fraction: 2.27 %	**Protein:** Total = 85.71g / p.s. = 21.43g **Fat:** Total = 73.37g / p.s. = 18.34g

45.   10 Minute Tandoori Salmon

When you're in a rush but need something flavor-packed for dinner, this will be your go-to recipe.

Ingredients

- 1 pound salmon (454g)
- 2 tsp of paprika (5g)
- 3 tsp mustard oil (14g)
- 1 tsp of coriander powder (1g)
- ¼ tsp ginger powder (1g)
- 1 tsp of garlic powder (3g)
- 1 tsp of chilli powder (3g)
- ½ tsp turmeric (2g)
- ½ tsp salt (3g)
- ½ tsp black pepper (2g)

Instructions

- Preheat oven to 425 F.
- Line a baking sheet with foil.
- Combine all spices in a bowl and mix well.
- Pour in the mustard oil. Beat to create a paste.
- Rub this paste on the salmon.
- Place the salmon on the baking sheet.
- Bake 4 to 6 minutes for every ½ inch of thickness.

Servings quantity: 2	Weight:
Energy (calories): Total = 738 kcal Per one serving = 369 kcal	Total = 485g Per one serving = 242.5g
Calorie breakdown: Protein: 54.5% / 403 kcal Fat: 42% / 309 kcal Carbohydrates: 3.5% / 27 kcal	**Total carbohydrate:** Total = 8.72g Per one serving = 4.36g
Carbohydrates mass fraction: 1.8%	**Protein:** Total = 95g / p.s. = 47.5g **Fat:** Total = 34.61g / p.s. = 17.30g

46.   Spinach Chicken

Looking for an easy dinner recipe when you're not in the mood to spend too much time in the kitchen? Try this.

Ingredients

- 2 ½ lb chicken cut into bite sized pieces (1134g)
- ½ bag of frozen spinach (142g)
- ½ pack of sliced mushrooms (113g)
- 1 medium onion (110g)
- basil (1g)
- butter (28g)
- garlic powder (10g)
- 1 lemon (58g)
- salt & pepper (23g)

Instructions

- Add butter to a large skillet.
- Add the chopped onion and mushrooms. sauté until onions are translucent.
- Mix well, then add the chopped chicken. Cook thoroughly.
- Add salt, pepper, basil and garlic powder to taste.
- Finally, add spinach and cook until wilted.
- Squeeze lemon juice on top and serve.

Servings quantity: 6	Weight:
Energy (calories): Total = 1581 kcal Per one serving = 263.5 kcal	Total = 1644g Per one serving = 274g
Calorie breakdown: Protein: 65% / 1022 kcal Fat: 27% / 430 kcal Carbohydrates: 8% / 131 kcal	**Total carbohydrate:** Total = 38.1g Per one serving = 6.35g
Carbohydrates mass fraction: 2.32%	**Protein:** Total = 244.5g / p.s. = 40.75g **Fat:** Total = 47.85g / p.s. = 7.98g

47.   Loaded cauliflower

One of the best low carb comfort foods ever!

Ingredients

- 2 slices of fried and crumbled bacon (23g)
- 1 lb cauliflower florets (454g)
- 4 oz of sour cream (113g)
- 2 tbsp of snipped chives (6g)
- 3 tbsp butter (43g)
- 1 cup grated cheddar cheese (113g)
- ¼ tsp garlic powder (1g)
- salt and pepper to taste (4g)

Instructions

- Cut the cauliflower into florets and put them in a bowl.
- Add 2 tbsp of water and microwave for 5 to 8 minutes.
- Drain the excess water and let sit uncovered until cool.
- Blend in a food processor until it gets fluffy.
- Add garlic powder, butter, sour cream. Blend until smooth.
- Place the mashed cauliflower in a fresh bowl, then add most of the chives.
- Add half of the cheddar cheese and season with salt and pepper.
- Top the loaded cauliflower with the remaining cheese, chives and bacon.
- Microwave for 2 to 3 minutes.

Servings quantity: 3	**Weight:**
Energy (calories): Total = 1145 kcal Per one serving = 381.67 kcal	Total = 756g Per one serving = 252g
Calorie breakdown: Protein: 16% / 182 kcal Fat: 73% / 840 kcal Carbohydrates: 11% / 125 kcal	**Total carbohydrate:** Total = 38.1g Per one serving = 6.35g
Carbohydrates mass fraction: 5.04%	**Protein:** Total = 48.4g / p.s. = 16.13g **Fat:** Total = 94.2g / p.s. = 31.4g

48. Keto Cheese Shell Taco Cups

Isn't the name cheesy enough to give this recipe a try?

Ingredients

For cheese cups

- 8 slices of your preferred cheese (239g)

For salsa

- 2 diced roma tomatoes (124g)
- 3 tbsp of diced red onion (30g)
- ½ finely diced fresh jalapeno (7g)
- 3 tbsp cilantro (3g)
- 1 tbsp lime juice (15g)

Instructions

- Preheat oven to 375 F.
- Line a baking sheet with parchment paper and place the cheese slices on it.
- Bake for 5 minutes.
- Remove the baking sheet and let cool slightly.
- Carefully remove the slices and place them in a muffin tin so they take on the cup's shape.
- Let them fully cool.

Making the salsa

- In a fresh bowl, add onions, roma tomatoes, cilantro, jalapenos and lime juice.
- Mix well.
- Place in the fridge for 30 minutes.
- Fill the cups with salsa filling and enjoy.

Servings quantity: 2 (4 cheese cups per serving)	Weight:
Energy (calories): Total = 876 kcal Per one serving = 438 kcal	Total = 403g Per one serving = 201.5g
Calorie breakdown: Protein: 27% / 238 kcal Fat: 68% / 599 kcal Carbohydrates: 4% / 39 kcal	**Total carbohydrate:** Total = 10.98g Per one serving = 5.49g
Carbohydrates mass fraction: 2.72%	**Protein:** Total = 56.45g / p.s. = 28.22g **Fat:** Total = 68.16g / p.s. = 34.08g

49.   Garlic Butter Brazilian Steak

Just 20 minutes to glory.

Ingredients

- 1 ½ lbs of steak, trimmed and cut evenly into 4 pieces (680g)
- 1 tbsp chopped fresh flat-leaf parsley (4g)
- 2 tbsp canola oil or vegetable oil (27g)
- 6 medium cloves of garlic (18g)
- 4 tbsp unsalted butter (56g)
- kosher salt (3g)
- freshly ground black pepper (1g)

Instructions

- Peel the garlic cloves then smash them using the side of your knife.
- Sprinkle the garlic with salt and mince it.
- Pat the steak dry, then season it slightly on both the sides with salt and pepper.
- Heat a heavy skillet on medium.
- Add the oil and heat until it begins to simmer.
- Add the steaks and brown on both sides.
- Transfer the steaks to a plate. Cover and rest.
- In an 8" skillet, melt butter on low heat.
- Add garlic and cook, tossing frequently until evenly golden in color.
- Slice the steaks and spoon the garlic butter on top.
- Garnish with parsley and serve.

Servings quantity: 4	**Weight:**
Energy (calories): Total = 1924 kcal Per one serving = 481 kcal	Total = 789g Per one serving = 197.25g
Calorie breakdown: Protein: 40% / 768 kcal Fat: 59% / 1144 kcal Carbohydrates: 1% / 25 kcal	**Total carbohydrate:** Total = 6.58g Per one serving = 1.65g
Carbohydrates mass fraction: 0.8%	**Protein:** Total = 192.52g / p.s. = 48.13g **Fat:** Total = 127.19g / p.s. = 31.8g

50.   Creamy cauliflower chowder

Once in awhile, it's just nice having soup for dinner, isn't it?

Ingredients

- 1 head of cauliflower cut into small florets (588g)
- ¾ cup diced carrots (96g)
- ½ cup diced onion (80g)
- 1 cup milk (244g)
- 1 tbsp butter (14g)
- ¼ cup cream cheese (58g)
- 5 cloves of minced garlic (15g)
- ½ tsp dried oregano (1g)
- 1 tsp freshly ground pepper (2g)
- salt to taste (6g)
- olive oil (14g) and 3 strips of cooked bacon (15g) for topping

Instructions

- Heat butter in a soup pot.
- Add onion and garlic and sauté for a few minutes.
- Add cauliflower, carrots, milk, pepper, salt, and oregano.
- Bring this mixture to boil and then reduce heat to a simmer.
- After the cauliflower is tender, remove from heat and pour the mixture into a blender.
- Blend soup until creamy then pour it back in the pot.
- Add a cup of water along with cream cheese.
- Simmer for 5 to 10 minutes and then turn off heat.
- Top with olive oil and bacon.

Servings quantity: 4	Weight:
Energy (calories): Total = 863 kcal Per one serving = 215.75 kcal	Total = 1133g Per one serving = 283.25g
Calorie breakdown: Protein: 10% / 87 kcal Fat: 61% / 522 kcal Carbohydrates: 29% / 253 kcal	**Total carbohydrate:** Total = 67.65g Per one serving = 16.91g
Carbohydrates mass fraction: 5.97%	**Protein:** Total = 27.15g / p.s. = 6.79g **Fat:** Total = 59.41g / p.s. = 14.85g

51.   Buttered Cod

A simple finale.

Ingredients

- 1 ½ lbs cod (680g)
- 6 tbsp unsalted butter (84g)

For the Seasoning-

- a few lemon slices (21g)
- ¼ tsp garlic powder (1g)
- ¾ tsp paprika (2g)
- ½ tsp salt (3g)
- ¼ tsp ground pepper (1g)
- herbs, parsley or cilantro (3g)

Instructions

- Mix all the seasoning ingredients in a small bowl.
- As desired, cut the cod into smaller pieces.
- Season with the mix.
- Melt butter in a large skillet on medium heat.
- Add the cod and cook for 2 minutes.
- Turn the cod, top with the leftover butter and continue cooking for 3 to 4 minutes.
- Drizzle with fresh lemon juice and serve.

Servings quantity: 2	Weight:
Energy (calories): Total = 905 kcal Per one serving = 452.5 kcal	Total = 795g Per one serving = 397.5g
Calorie breakdown: Protein: 50% / 457 kcal Fat: 49% / 445 kcal Carbohydrates: 1% / 11 kcal	**Total carbohydrate:** Total = 4.08g Per one serving = 2.04g
Carbohydrates mass fraction: 0.5%	**Protein:** Total = 107.45g / p.s. = 53.73g **Fat:** Total = 49.41g / p.s. = 24.71g

Conversion Table

Equivalents

U.S.	U.S.
16 tablespoons	1 cup
12 tablespoons	3/4 cup
10 tablespoons + 2 teaspoons	2/3 cup
8 tablespoons	1/2 cup
6 tablespoons	3/8 cup
5 tablespoons + 1 teaspoon	1/3 cup
4 tablespoons	1/4 cup
2 tablespoons + 2 teaspoons	1/6 cup
2 tablespoons	1/8 cup
1 tablespoon	1/16 cup
1 pint	2 cups
1 quart	2 pints
1 tablespoon	3 teaspoons
1 cup	48 teaspoons
1 cup	16 tablespoons

Capacity

U.S.	METRIC
1/5 teaspoon	1 ml
1 teaspoon (tsp)	5 ml
1 tablespoon (tbsp)	15 ml
1 fluid oz.	30 ml
1/5 cup	50 ml
1/4 cup	60 ml
1/3 cup	80 ml
3.4 fluid oz.	100 ml
1/2 cup	120 ml
2/3 cup	160 ml
3/4 cup	180 ml
1 cup	240 ml
1 pint (2 cups)	480 ml
1 quart (4 cups)	.95 liter
34 fluid oz.	1 liter
4.2 cups	1 liter
2.1 pints	1 liter
1.06 quarts	1 liter
.26 gallon	1 liter
4 quarts (1 gallon)	3.8 liters

Weight

U.S.	METRIC
.035 ounce	1 gram
0.5 oz.	14 grams
1 oz.	28 grams
1/4 pound (lb)	113 grams
1/3 pound (lb)	151 grams
1/2 pound (lb)	227 grams
1 pound (lb)	454 grams
1.10 pounds (lbs)	500 grams
2.205 pounds (lbs)	1 kilogram
35 oz.	1 kilogram

Flour kinds comparative table

Serv.size: 1 cup	Calories	Carbs	Protein	Fat	Weight
Almond flour	640 kcal	20 g	24 g	56 g	100 g
Hazelnut flour	720 kcal	20 g	16 g	68 g	95 g
Coconut flour	480 kcal	64 g	16 g	16 g	115 g
Chickpea flour	440 kcal	72 g	24 g	8 g	90 g
Amaranth flour	440 kcal	80 g	16 g	8 g	108 g
Rice flour	580 kcal	128 g	8.8 g	2.4 g	150 g

Conclusion

Now that you have these recipes, are you all set to follow a ketogenic diet? With so much diversity, keto shouldn't be a hassle whatsoever.

You can mix and match these recipes and explore other options. Variety will keep your palate entertained and your cravings in check. Keep in mind the amount of calories you're consuming, especially from carbs. With a small amount of effort and some persistence, your adherence to a ketogenic diet will result in increased health, vitality, and significant weight loss in a relatively brief period of time.

We know losing weight isn't an easy task and there are plenty of dieting mistakes you have, and can, make. When you opt for keto, you'll be able to shed pounds in a systematic manner while retaining lean muscle mass and without depriving yourself of good food.

We hope you follow these recipes and see how useful (and tasty!) they are.

Dear Reader,

Thank you again for purchasing this book!
I hope this book was helpful for you.

Finally, if you enjoyed this book, I'd highly appreciate if you make a favor and leave a review for this book on Amazon.

The opinion of every reader is very important for me. It helps me to make my books better and more useful.

Also, your review will be really useful for other customers! Most of the customers consider reviews are the most important factors which can help them to choose a book.

To leave a review, you can just go to the link or scan QR-code:
https://www.amazon.com/Keto-Diet-Beginners-Ketogenic-Cookbook/dp/1522000690/#customerReviews

The process only takes a minute or so.

Thanks in advance for your time, and thanks again for choosing my book.

And, please, don't forget to receive your free bonus on the next page.

I wish you all the best.

Sincerely yours,
Amanda Lee

REMINDER:

Get Your Free Bonus

I wanted to show my appreciation that you support my work so I've put together a bonus for you.

Keto Diet for Beginners:

Ketogenic Smoothie and Dessert Recipes

Just visit the link or scan QR-code to download it now:

https://wondergoodsfactory.com/landing-pages/amanda-lee-free-bonus-download/

Thanks!

Amanda Lee